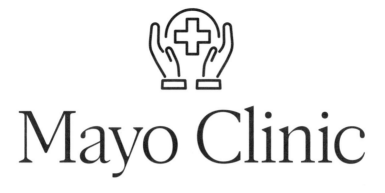

Mayo Clinic

GUIDE TO

Holistic Health

UNLOCK YOUR BODY'S
NATURAL HEALING POWERS

BRENT A. BAUER, M.D.

 Press

MAYO CLINIC PRESS

Medical Editor | Brent A. Bauer, M.D.

Publisher | Daniel J. Harke

Editor in Chief | Nina E. Wiener

Managing Editor | Rachel A. Haring Bartony

Art Director | Stewart J. Koski

Production Design | Amanda J. Knapp

Illustration and Photography | Mayo Clinic Media Support Services

Editorial Research Librarian | Morgan T. Wentworth, M.L.S.

Contributors | Roberto P. Benzo, M.D. | Lynn Borkenhagen | Tony Y. Chon, M.D. | Ivana T. Croghan, Ph.D. | Susanne M. Cutshall, APRN, CNS, D.N.P., M.S. | Alexander Do, L.Ac. | Debbie L. Fuehrer, M.A., L.P.C.C. | Jennifer L. Hauschulz, BCTMB | Benjamin D. Holmes, D.C., Ph.D. | Linda Huang, Pharm.D., R.Ph., BCPS | Ryan T. Hurt, M.D., Ph.D. | Stephen Kopecky, M.D. | Molly J. Mallory, L.Ac. | Abbey K. Metzger, D.N.P., R.N., CHPN | Denise M. Millstine, M.D. | Michael R. Mueller, M.D. | Steven W. Ressler, M.D. | Whitney M. Romine | Jon C. Tilburt, M.D. | Ann Vincent, M.D. | Jenna G. Whiting | Lina Zeldovich

Image Credits | All photographs and illustrations are copyright of Mayo Foundation for Medical Education and Research (MFMER), except for the following: COVER, CREDIT: Yaremchuk Diana/iStock / Getty Images Plus via Getty Images; rambo182 / DigitalVision Vectors via Getty Images; appleuzr / DigitalVision Vectors via Getty Images; bounward / DigitalVision Vectors via Getty Images | p. 52, CREDIT: AlexeyBlogoodf/ iStock / Getty Images via Getty Images | p. 52, 53, 71, 82, 88, 96, 111, 116, 128, 136, 141, 156, 159, 165, 168, 171, 180, 184, 187, 190, 193, 198, 205, 207, 213, 219, 220, 223, CREDIT: appleuzr / DigitalVision Vectors via Getty Images | p. 100, 105, CREDIT: Aleksandr Kharitonov / iStock / Getty Images via Getty Image

When you purchase Mayo Clinic newsletters and books, proceeds are used to further medical education and research at Mayo Clinic. You not only get answers to your questions on health, you become part of the solution.

Published by Mayo Clinic Press

© 2024 Mayo Foundation for Medical Education and Research (MFMER)

MAYO, MAYO CLINIC and the Mayo triple-shield logo are marks of Mayo Foundation for Medical Education and Research. All rights reserved. No part of this book may be reproduced, stored in a retrieval system, or transmitted, in any form or by any means, electronic, mechanical, photocopying, recording or otherwise, without the prior written permission of the publisher.

The information in this book is true and complete to the best of our knowledge. This book is intended only as an informative guide for those wishing to learn more about health issues. It is not intended to replace, countermand or conflict with advice given to you by your own physician. The ultimate decision concerning your care should be made between you and your doctor. Information in this book is offered with no guarantees. The author and publisher disclaim all liability in connection with the use of this book.

For bulk sales to employers, member groups and health-related companies, contact Mayo Clinic, 200 First St. SW, Rochester, MN 55905, or send an email to **SpecialSalesMayoBooks@mayo.edu.**

To stay informed about Mayo Clinic Press, please subscribe to our free e-newsletter at **MCPress.MayoClinic.org** or follow us on social media.

ISBN 979-8-88770-240-7 hardcover
ISBN 979-8-88770-291-9 ebook

Library of Congress Control Number: 2023948916

Printed in the United States of America

contents

6 Preface

PART 1 | A HOLISTIC APPROACH TO HEALTH

---

12 HEALTH IS MORE THAN MEDICINE
13 The link between mind and body
15 Whole health
16 Maximizing wellness
17 Putting it into practice

20 WHOLE-HEALTH FUNDAMENTALS
21 Exercise
25 Sleep
28 Nutrition
34 Stress management
38 Social connectedness
43 Spirituality and purpose
45 Connection with nature

50 WELLNESS DURING ILLNESS
51 Putting your innate healing powers to work
56 Balancing medicine and wellness
57 Living well despite discomfort or pain
60 Looking ahead

PART 2 | THERAPIES A–Z

64	Acupuncture	163	Music therapy
73	Animal-assisted services	167	Naturopathy
80	Aromatherapy	170	Pilates
86	Art therapy	173	Probiotics
90	Biofeedback	179	Progressive muscle relaxation
98	Cannabis and cannabinoids	182	Psychedelics
106	Cryotherapy	186	Qigong
109	Deep breathing	190	Reflexology
113	Guided imagery	193	Reiki
116	Healing touch	197	Rolfing
119	Herbs and supplements	199	Saunas
126	Homeopathy	202	Spinal manipulation
131	Hot tubs and warm pools	209	Tai chi
134	Hypnotherapy	213	*Tui na* / Chinese massage
139	Massage therapy	216	Virtual reality
148	Meditation and mindfulness	218	Yoga
158	Multivitamins		

PART 3 | TOOL KIT

226	Assess your health and set your goals	236	Partnering with your healthcare team
232	5 steps for moving forward	238	Finding high-quality research
233	Holistic health on a budget	243	Transforming your health and your future

244 **Additional resources**

246 **Index**

Preface

What does the word *whole* mean to you? Depending on the dictionary, it's often defined as "all of something." In other words, it includes everything about something, not just a particular part or piece. The term *holism* has a similar meaning: the view that an integrated whole stands for more than just the sum of its parts.

So, what does it mean when the word *holistic* is used in relation to health? At its most basic level, it means considering the person as a whole — mind, body and spirit. The focus isn't just on a specific part, such as the heart, but on how the heart fits in with the rest of the body, and how the rest of the body impacts the heart. It also means considering how a person's emotions, lifestyle, relationships, stressors, resources and spirituality impact the health of the heart — and how these aspects may be impacted by heart health as well.

The word *health* means different things to different people. One definition I like is provided by the World Health Organization: "Health is a state of complete physical, mental and social well-being and not merely the absence of disease or infirmity." This definition emphasizes the importance of looking at the person's whole health.

Modern medicine has become extremely successful at treating many types of diseases, allowing people to live much longer than they might otherwise. When our bodies are broken, modern medicine can provide miraculous interventions to help restore them. But there's also a growing realization that high-tech medicine by itself may not be enough to truly promote our well-being.

A person who receives a stent to treat a blocked artery that caused a heart attack has had the emergency addressed. But what about factors that might have led to the heart attack in the first place? These might include obvious factors, such as high cholesterol and smoking — and modern medicine usually has a plan to help people work on addressing these kinds of measurable risk factors. But what about the role of stress? Or loneliness? Here, science offers few answers, if any.

In an era of efficiency and urgent care systems, there is little time for holistic medicine. Modern health professionals rarely have more than a few minutes with each person to make sure that important lifestyle factors — such as nutrition, exercise, emotional health, sleep, community, spirituality and access to nature — are fully explored and implemented in the best way for that person.

The truth is, if we want to approach our own health in a holistic way, we need to take ownership of it. That means it's up to each of us to know what we need to reach a complete state of well-being — mind, body and spirit.

My colleagues in Integrative Medicine and Health at Mayo Clinic and I developed this book to help you explore all aspects of your personal health. The book covers a broad range of topics; some may sound quite familiar, and others may be new to you. You may be successful in some areas already, and discover other areas where you recognize the opportunity for change.

Since each person is unique, no two readers will take away the same message or plan from this book. For that reason, this book isn't meant to be a step-by-step guide. Instead, we hope it provides you with a general blueprint that addresses the key domains of holistic health, with some strategies within each for you to explore. We also want to give you an evidence-based starting point for you to begin asking the deep questions about what you need to do to optimize your health.

With this foundation, we encourage you to reach out to your primary care team and invite them to be a part of your journey. If you incorporate new members into your whole healthcare team — such as an acupuncturist, massage therapist or life coach — let your primary care team know. And encourage all of your care team members to communicate so that they can help you achieve the best possible integrated approach to your holistic health.

HOW TO USE THIS RESOURCE

This book is intended to provide you with straightforward information about taking a holistic approach to your health. We want you to know about the various therapies we use, as well as other ones in common use, and the science and evidence about their use. We also included some emerging therapies that may prove helpful as more evidence accumulates.

First, you'll learn about lifestyle strategies that can help you build a solid foundation and how these strategies can help ensure that you get the most out of the efforts you're making to improve your health. You'll also discover how to maximize your health even when — or especially when — you're managing a chronic illness or other condition.

In the "Therapies A–Z" section, you'll find a list of specific therapies that are often used as part of a holistic approach to maximizing health and quality of life. In our discussion of each treatment, you'll learn about the latest research, the safety and effectiveness of the product or practice, and any potential risks.

Finally, we've included a practical information tool kit to help you get started on your own holistic health journey. Here you can take steps to assess your health, set goals and find ways to incorporate holistic health approaches into your everyday life that work for you.

We hope that the *Mayo Clinic Guide to Holistic Health* will serve as your personal guide to enjoying all aspects of your health to the fullest.

Brent A. Bauer, M.D.

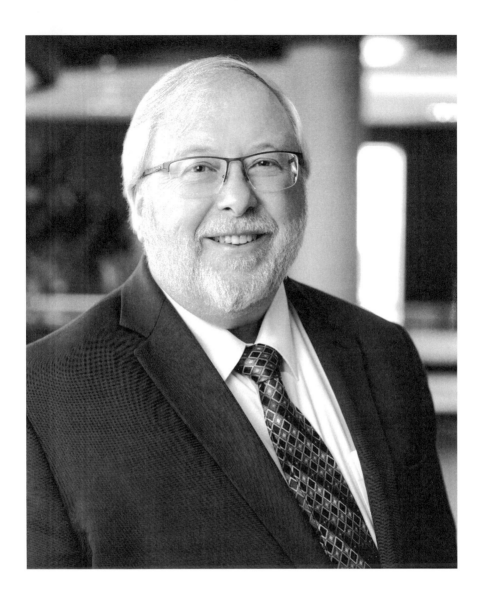

Brent A. Bauer, M.D., is board certified in internal medicine. He is the research chair for Mayo Clinic Integrative Medicine and Health and a doctor in the Division of General Internal Medicine. He is also a professor of medicine at Mayo Clinic College of Medicine and Science. Dr. Bauer focuses on the scientific evaluation of integrative medicine therapies. He has served as medical director of Rejuvenate, the first spa at Mayo Clinic, and of the Well Living Lab, a collaboration between Delos and Mayo Clinic that is exploring the impact of the indoor environment on wellness.

PART 1

A holistic approach to health

Health is more than medicine

It's Wednesday night and Roberto P. Benzo, M.D., founding director of the Mindful Breathing Laboratory at Mayo Clinic in Rochester, Minnesota, is starting a virtual meditation session. As he accepts requests to join, more and more squares fill up his screen. People are joining from all over the place — some from Minnesota, others from Arizona and Florida. Some of them are Mayo Clinic patients, recovering from surgeries or illnesses, some are caregivers, and others are Mayo Clinic nurses and staff.

As he begins, Dr. Benzo speaks to his listeners in a calming, soothing voice, coaxing them to sit back, relax and be mindful of their bodies, their breathing and what's happening right now. "Observe the movie of your life in the present moment and try to not like or dislike it," he says. "Just sit and feel your body moving as you breathe in and breathe out, and be completely aware of the things that are in your mind and in your heart."

As he speaks, a sense of calm seems to travel over the distance, reaching the attendees. On the screen, participants snuggle in their chairs, getting more comfortable. Some close their eyes and lie back. One person cuddles up with a big, fluffy brown cat. Dr. Benzo keeps talking, suggesting that listeners stay in the present moment, letting their thoughts go.

"It's best to relinquish thoughts and stop passing judgments," he adds, but those whose speedy minds are going too fast shouldn't punish themselves for thinking too much. "Your meditation is just observing that speedy mind," Dr. Benzo says. He goes on: "This practice allows you to observe everything in your body, particularly if you're suffering from something, your emotions, your urges, desires, thoughts. Just keep observing, detaching yourself from the idea of being sick or emotional. We are beyond that; we're completely in the present, completely in the 'now.'" And that state can be very healing, he notes. "We have the willingness to fix anything."

THE LINK BETWEEN MIND AND BODY

Most ancient healing practices, such as traditional Chinese medicine and Indian Ayurvedic medicine, have long held that the mind and body are closely linked. Modern science is bringing a new perspective to this connection.

A groundbreaking brain-imaging study published in 2023 demonstrated how the many functions of the mind and body are interwoven. The study showed that the parts of the brain that control movement are tightly meshed with the networks responsible for conscious efforts, such as thinking and planning, as well as involuntary ones such as heartbeat and blood pressure. The findings suggest that the perceptions of the mind are literally linked to the actions of the body.

Other research has shown that the mind can have a powerful influence on the body. Chronic mental stress directly affects not only our emotional wellness but our physical health as well. When we are distressed, especially for extended periods of time, it dampens our immune system response, lowering our resilience and making us more vulnerable to a long list of health problems. Chronic stress, for example, can increase levels of molecules called pro-inflammatory cytokines, an overabundance of which contributes to chronic inflammation and illnesses such as heart disease, type 2 diabetes and some types of cancer.

The body, and physical ailments that affect it, also can affect the mind. For example, evidence indicates that people who have diabetes are 2 to 3 times more likely to be depressed, and people who have chronic pain often experience anxiety.

As science continues to reveal the complex interactions between mind states and bodily functions, there's a growing recognition that good health means more than just addressing the physical aspects of disease. Although modern medicine can effectively treat many illnesses, it's not a cure-all. In addition, medical treatments often come with side effects, which can themselves be damaging.

Interest in a more holistic approach to healthcare is growing. In the medical field, this approach is known as integrative medicine (see page 14), a type of healthcare that seeks to treat the whole person, not just the person's disease or condition. It involves evidence-informed approaches to managing mental factors such as stress and anxiety that can impact other aspects of health, including disease symptoms.

It's not possible to wish cancer away or think hard enough to make diabetes disappear, but it is possible to manage your thoughts and train your mind to develop a more intentional focus. And by doing so, you can address worries and even create new pathways in your brain that help you experience less stress and anger. Experiencing fewer negative thoughts and emotions makes room for a more positive mindset and more meaningful actions, all of which can facilitate healthy habits, ease the burden of disease on your body and make your overall quality of life better.

WHAT IS INTEGRATIVE MEDICINE?

According to the Academic Consortium for Integrative Medicine & Health, integrative medicine is a form of healthcare that focuses on the whole person, is informed by evidence, and makes use of all appropriate therapeutic and lifestyle approaches, healthcare professionals and disciplines to achieve optimal health and healing.

Integrative medicine professionals work with your healthcare team to provide you with a comprehensive health plan. For example, integrative therapies are used to help people with medical conditions — such as cancer, chonic fatigue or chronic pain — feel better by reducing fatigue, nausea, pain and anxiety.

But integrative medicine isn't just about treating illness; it's about helping you maintain your health in the first place. And in many cases it means bringing new therapies and approaches to the table. An integrative approach helps lead you into a complete lifestyle of wellness.

To date, over 75 academic medical centers have joined the Academic Consortium for Integrative Medicine & Health. Members include Mayo Clinic, Duke University, Harvard Medical School and many other institutions in the United States and abroad. The mission of this organization is to advance the principles and practices of integrative medicine.

Mayo Clinic Integrative Medicine and Health is a dedicated program within the clinic that offers a range of services, including many of the therapies discussed in this book. It also offers wellness coaching, as well as stress management and resilience training.

WHOLE HEALTH

Our physical bodies are important, but so are our minds, emotions, social connections, cultural traditions, stories, and hopes and dreams. These aspects of ourselves are deeply intertwined. Each plays an important role in overall health.

Making the most of your health involves taking a proactive, holistic approach to healthcare that aims to increase your quality of life and prevent illness by addressing all aspects of your life. Yes, this means regular health screenings, early detection of health problems and preventive measures to address risk factors before they become serious health issues. But it also means recognizing that health is a dynamic process that requires ongoing attention and effort, and that small lifestyle changes can have a big impact on overall health and well-being.

Having a good quality of life implies living your life fully — and enjoying it. Rather than asking "What's the matter with you?" and focusing on problems that manifest themselves physically, a holistic approach to health asks, "What matters to you?" Then the next question becomes, "How do you apply that knowledge to your daily decisions?"

EXPERT INSIGHT
PATIENT CENTERED

Integrative medicine has gone by several different names over the years, all aiming to describe something that is separate from conventional medicine. But it's much more than that. It's an open-minded, patient-centered pragmatism about whole-person health.

Increasingly, healthcare organizations are seeing integrative medicine as a way to help prevent chronic disease and promote good health. A report from the National Academy of Medicine suggests that integrative health — using the best, evidence-informed approaches to care — can empower each one of us to build our own wellness plan and partner with our healthcare teams to put it into action.

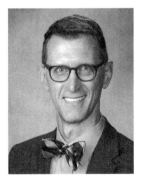

Jon C. Tilburt, M.D.
General Internal Medicine

MAXIMIZING WELLNESS

Instead of viewing healthcare as something that happens at the doctor's office, think of it as a personalized approach to wellness that enables you to become the most resilient and healthy person you can be. This includes nourishing the body, engaging the mind, nurturing the spirit, managing stress and engaging with others socially.

Physical wellness

Physical wellness means enjoying a thriving lifestyle. This involves eating healthy foods, getting enough sleep, being active and minimizing risky behaviors such as drinking or smoking. For some, it requires managing chronic health conditions or overcoming a disease.

Intellectual wellness

Intellectual wellness is about engaging in mentally stimulating and creative activities. It is the ability to think critically, reason objectively, make responsible decisions and explore new ideas and different points of view. These skills can span from your personal life to your work life. For many people, being in a healthy state of mind requires a meaningful career that brings fulfillment and satisfaction. People who thrive intellectually enjoy learning, stay curious and feel confident in themselves.

Spiritual wellness

Spiritual wellness is about having a meaning and purpose in life, as well as engaging in practices that reflect one's beliefs, values, morals and ethics. It may or may not involve religious activities. Research finds that people who feel they have purpose live longer and healthier lives. A spiritually well person devotes time to gratitude and self-reflection, practices acceptance and forgiveness, and cultivates compassion and respect for others.

Emotional wellness

Emotional wellness is about being able to experience and appropriately express a wide range of emotions, from humor to joy to fear and from anger to frustration to sadness. It also includes being able to be assertive when necessary and able to handle confrontations. Staying well emotionally includes self-esteem, self-acceptance and the ability to experience and cope with feelings. People who are well emotionally tend to be optimistic, to be resilient and to cope well with stress.

Social wellness

Social wellness is about connecting with your friends and family circles as well as your community. Being well at a social level means that you can forge friendships and close relationships, and are accepting of others and enjoy their company. That might involve being mindful of your own heritage as well as appreciating the diversity of other people's social, cultural and religious backgrounds.

PUTTING IT INTO PRACTICE

As Dr. Benzo's session comes to an end, he asks participants if they want to share how they feel. The consensus is that they feel calmer and more relaxed than before. Some share that they also feel more positive and optimistic. Others add that they feel refreshed and have a sense of gratitude. Several note that they feel more strength to cope. Their minds generated positive emotions, which impacted their physiological states. Dr. Benzo's meditation session illustrates the value of using a practice such as meditation as part of a holistic health approach. It's not magic or a miracle cure, but it helps the people participating to actively care for themselves and focus on what matters to them.

Today, more and more physicians are introducing new therapies and approaches into their practice — such as meditation, tai chi, and yoga — to enhance their patients' wellness in a multitude of ways. Adding these practices to mainstream medical therapies, a practice also known as integrative medicine (see page 14), allows medical professionals to treat people holistically, according to what each may need.

As medicine shifts toward wellness and disease prevention, holistic practices play an important role in healthcare. In this holistic approach to health, you are the key ingredient — you have inherent wisdom about what is right for you. You are the captain of your healthcare team, partnering with medical professionals to chart your own personalized, self-care course — and alter it as necessary to make the most of your life.

INTEGRATIVE VS. ALTERNATIVE: WHAT'S THE DIFFERENCE?

Alternative medicine is used *in place of* conventional medicine. An example of an alternative therapy is using a special diet to treat cancer in place of undergoing surgery, radiation or chemotherapy that has been recommended by a conventional doctor.

Integrative medicine, on the other hand, *combines* mainstream medical treatments and complementary therapies that have scientific evidence of their safety and efficacy. An example of an integrative therapy is using acupuncture to help lessen nausea after surgery.

Health is more than medicine

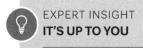

EXPERT INSIGHT
IT'S UP TO YOU

Stephen Kopecky, M.D., tells his patients that they have a new part-time job: taking care of their own health. "No one in the world cares about your health more than you do," he says. If you won't focus on your health, no one else will.

"There are a lot of institutions that care about your *illness*," Dr. Kopecky adds — but that's different. "They will gladly treat you. They'll do stents, they'll put in devices, they'll do surgeries, but they don't really care about your *health* because they're not paid to keep you in good health."

Keeping yourself in good health physically, mentally and spiritually falls on you. Staying strong, energetic and resilient takes your own efforts too. "I've been telling this to all my patients, especially since the pandemic," Dr. Kopecky says.

Pandemic effects
The COVID-19 pandemic took a huge toll on people's health — and not just because of the virus. The pandemic changed what and how we eat, how we live and connect with others, and the amount of time we spend being active. To cope with added stress, anxiety and uncertainty during the pandemic, people resorted to pajamas, comfort foods and binge-watching TV. That was quite understandable. But when COVID-19 abated, some of these new habits, often less healthy, didn't go away.

"In the beginning of the pandemic, a little over 50% of our calories came from ultraprocessed foods, which have too much salt, too much sugar, too much fat and too many calories in them," says Dr. Kopecky. "And now that the pandemic is over, we're getting almost 60% of our calories from ultraprocessed foods. In the beginning of the pandemic, we were eating about 3.5 grams of sodium a day. And now we are eating about 4 grams a day, while we should eat only about 2 grams." As a society, we grew accustomed to the ease of processed foods and ordering meals in, so now we just continue.

We also became far more sedentary because we got used to moving less. Many of us still work from home, at least part of the week. That means that we don't walk to a bus or a train or even to a parking lot anymore. Nor do we go out to lunch or coffee breaks with our coworkers and colleagues.

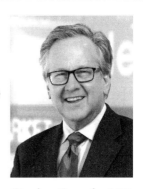

Stephen Kopecky, M.D.
Cardiovascular Medicine

We got used to ordering takeout from restaurants online, as well as groceries, clothes, books, shoes, household items and everything else. It is undoubtedly more convenient to order an item online than to go out shopping for it.

Before the pandemic, people may have gone to a mall or shopping center, where they would spend a few hours walking around, but the pandemic reshaped many societal habits. "Our activity level has gone down to nothing," Dr. Kopecky points out. "And while we sit at home, we also have more access to foods and snacks."

To change, start small
Humans are creatures of habit. Habits are hard to break, particularly the unhealthy ones, because many of them give us comfort. Dr. Kopecky recommends not breaking bad habits but rather replacing them with better ones. For example, you can start with something small such as taking a walk after dinner rather than watching a show. Or you can switch from snacking on chips to snacking on carrots and sweet peppers. Taking small initial steps will add up and gradually improve your wellness levels.

Some bad habits form because of too much stress, high workload or living with chronic illness. Some of these life factors can't be removed, but you can alter your response to them and boost your overall resilience to deal with them better. That will likely also improve your health, wellness and overall quality of life — in a holistic way.

Whole-health fundamentals

One of the key principles of a holistic health approach is a focus on the whole person. No treatment or therapy — conventional or complementary — can help you reach your health goals if you don't take steps to build your foundation of wellness first.

The basic components of a healthy life — exercise, sleep, nutrition, stress management, a strong support network, a sense of purpose and a connection with the natural world — provide your wellness foundation. No complementary therapy can take the place of these basic tenets of personal wellness. And without these basics, medical interventions may not work as well.

As you embark on your journey toward better health, start with these fundamentals. Often you'll find they overlap, lending themselves very well to holistic living. For example, going for a walk outside lets you exercise *and* connect with nature. Eating a healthy dinner with friends you really connect with benefits your body *and* your spirit.

In addition, many of the complementary therapies and techniques in the "Therapies A–Z" section can help you reduce stress, sleep better and improve your balance and muscle tone. Every step you take to improve your personal wellness is a step toward living a longer, more holistic and more enjoyable life.

But first, the basics. Here are the seven key domains that make up whole-health wellness.

EXERCISE

Exercise is probably the single most important thing you can do to live well. Even in moderate amounts, exercise can help you better enjoy life and prevent disease. By introducing a moderate amount of physical activity into your daily life, you can significantly improve your overall health, well-being and quality of life. The activity you choose to do is up to you, but try to include both aerobic activity and resistance training. And keep in mind: The more you exercise, the more you may benefit.

Benefits of exercise

Whether you're 25 or 85, regular repetitive physical activity can provide the benefits you need to help you look and feel better and enjoy great health.

Anti-inflammatory effects

Regular exercise helps keep inflammation in check. When you move about, your muscles contract, stimulating an anti-inflammatory response set in motion by your immune system. This reduces circulation of pro-inflammatory compounds, such as interleukins and cytokines, in the bloodstream — elements that can damage the lining of your arteries, resulting in stiff artery walls, formation of plaques and increased blood pressure. Regular exercise also reduces chronic inflammation that contributes to DNA damage, thus helping to prevent changes that could lead to cancer.

Insulin benefits

Physical activity, especially resistance training, keeps your body sensitive to the effects of insulin, the hormone that regulates blood sugar levels. You want your cells to be receptive to insulin so that you don't have high levels of the hormone traveling through your bloodstream. Too much insulin can lead to inflammation and damage the lining of your arteries. This is what happens with type 2 diabetes.

Effects on weight and muscle mass

When you take part in physical activity, you burn calories. The more intense the activity, the more calories you burn. Burning calories helps prevent excess weight gain and helps maintain weight lost through dietary changes. Because exercise helps you reach and maintain a healthy weight, it reduces the risks and complications of diseases and conditions associated with being overweight, such as sleep apnea and type 2 diabetes.

Regular exercise — particularly resistance training — strengthens your muscles and slows the loss of muscle mass as you age. It also keeps bones strong by maintaining bone density, which plays an important role in preventing bone diseases such as osteoporosis.

Whole-health fundamentals **21**

Heart and lung health

Being active boosts high-density lipoprotein (HDL) cholesterol, the "good" cholesterol, and it decreases unhealthy triglycerides. This one-two punch keeps your blood flowing smoothly, which lowers your risk of cardiovascular

THE RISKS OF BEING SEDENTARY

Our bodies are designed to run, jump and manipulate objects. But how often do we use our bodies at their full potential? With today's lifestyle, not very often. In fact, we've made being sedentary into a new norm. We get aggravated by a broken elevator that pushes us to walk up the stairs, or we drive around a retailer's parking lot to find the spot nearest the entrance rather than walk a few extra feet. Many of us sit at a desk throughout the workday and then relax by once again sitting and scrolling through digital media, reading a book, or watching TV.

This excessive amount of sitting is a fairly new phenomenon. Early humans moved a lot. They walked long distances while foraging, periodically chased prey or ran away from predators, and used their strength for other daily activities. When humans turned to farming, they worked in the fields, cut wood, built homes and shepherded animals. Even 200 years ago, 90% of people still lived in agricultural communities. People sat for 3 to 5 hours per day, but only to take breaks from working. In comparison, modern Americans sit for 13 to 15 hours per day.

For over 10 years, physical inactivity has been recognized as a global problem with widespread health, economic and social impacts. In a 2022 national survey, more than a quarter of Americans reported that outside of their regular job, they had not engaged in any physical activity in the previous month, be it walking, golfing or gardening. Less than 30% of responders living in metropolitan areas met physical activity guidelines. And even fewer people living outside of metropolitan areas did so — slightly over 16%. Globally, 1 in 4 adults don't meet the recommended levels of physical activity.

Unfortunately, our bodies weren't built to deal with so much inactivity. Leading a mostly sedentary lifestyle has been linked to many diseases and conditions, including obesity, hypertension, back pain, cancer, cardiovascular disease and depression. On the other hand, moving around — walking, playing, exercising and engaging in general physical activity — has many benefits (see page 21).

diseases. Exercise also sends oxygen and nutrients to your tissues and helps your heart and lungs work more efficiently. And when your heart and lung health improve, you have more energy and greater stamina.

Mental and emotional well-being
Exercise stimulates the production of endorphins, brain chemicals that produce feelings of well-being and can help fight depression. Daytime exercise and physical activity also can help you sleep better.

Focusing on physical motion helps to calm your mind and relieve stress. You also tend to feel better about yourself when you exercise regularly, which can boost your confidence and improve your self-esteem.

> **BEFORE YOU START AN EXERCISE PROGRAM**
>
> Remember to check with your healthcare team before starting a new exercise program, especially if you have any concerns about your fitness or haven't exercised for a long time. Also check with a healthcare professional if you have chronic health problems, such as heart disease, diabetes or arthritis.

Design your fitness program

Being fit means different things to different people. Perhaps it means you're comfortable with your body, your balance and your strength. Or it may mean doing the activities you want to without discomfort. Or that your heart rate slows to a healthy level, and your blood pressure and blood sugar are well managed. Following are key types of exercise that are intended to help you become more physically fit. Keep in mind that everyone is built differently and has different motivations when it comes to physical fitness. Consider finding a daily activity you like to do and work from there.

Aerobic fitness
Aerobic activity, also known as cardio or endurance activity, is the core of most fitness training programs. Aerobic exercise is any activity that causes you to breathe faster and more deeply, which sends more oxygen to your blood. Your heart will beat faster, which sends more blood flow to your muscles and back to your lungs. The greater your aerobic fitness, the more efficiently your heart, lungs and blood vessels carry oxygen throughout your body.

Each week, most adults should aim for at least 150 minutes of moderate-intensity aerobic activity, 75 minutes of vigorous aerobic activity or a

Whole-health fundamentals 23

combination of the two. You can break up activity into shorter periods of exercise and aim to move more during the day. Even if you don't hit these goals, any amount is better than none at all.

To get more training out of a short amount of time, try high-intensity interval training, also called HIIT. HIIT involves doing short bursts of intense activity of around 30 seconds interposed with recovery periods of lighter activity for around 1 to 2 minutes. So you can switch between brisk walking and relaxed walking, for example. Or add bursts of jogging during your brisk walks. You can get in the same cardiovascular shape with interval training as you would with traditional training, but with less time spent exercising.

Strength training

Strength training is another key part of a fitness training plan. Aim to train all the major muscle groups at least twice a week.

Most gyms offer many resistance machines, free weights and other strength training tools. But you don't need to be a gym member or buy costly equipment to get strength training benefits.

Handheld weights or homemade weights, such as plastic soft drink bottles filled with water or sand, may work just as well. Or use low-cost resistance bands. Your own body weight counts too. Try pushups, pullups, situps and leg squats.

Core exercises

The muscles in the stomach area, lower back and pelvis are known as the core muscles. Core exercises help you train the muscles to support the spine in your back. And they help you use your upper and lower body muscles more effectively. So what counts as a core exercise? A core exercise is any exercise that uses the trunk of the body without support. Some core exercises are bridges, planks, situps and fitness ball exercises.

Balance training

Balance exercises stabilize core muscles and can help you keep your balance. Especially as you get older, balance exercises can help prevent falls and keep you doing things on you own. Try standing on one leg for longer periods of time to improve your stability. Activities such as tai chi (see page 209) can boost balance too.

Flexibility and stretching

Flexibility is an important piece of physical fitness. Being more flexible can make it easier for you to do many everyday activities. Stretching exercises can help increase flexibility. They also can improve the range of motion of your joints and help with better posture. Regular stretching can help lessen stress and tension. Try to stretch each time you exercise. Stretch after you work out when your muscles are warm and open to stretching. Try to hold your stretches for at least 30 seconds. If you don't exercise often, try to stretch at least 2 or 3 times a week after warming up to keep flexible. Activities such as yoga help you stay flexible too.

SLEEP

Sleep is vital for good health and well-being. If you're not getting enough shut-eye regularly, you're increasing your risk of developing unhealthy conditions.

When you sleep, your body deploys its natural ability to heal itself, clear away toxins and process memories. Sleep is an essential function that enables you to recharge, restore and regenerate. It is also important for your metabolism, immunity and other body functions and systems that help fight off disease.

The night shift

Although sleep is a basic biological process, what happens during sleep is actually quite complex. When you sleep, your body takes on the "night shift," flowing through different stages that repeat several times throughout the period of sleep. While you slumber, your brain stays active, cycling through two distinct phases: rapid eye movement (REM) sleep and non-REM sleep. Some of these stages help you feel rested and energetic when you wake up. Other stages enable you to learn information and form memories.

Throughout the night, your breathing, heart rate and blood pressure rise and fall, cycles that are important for cardiovascular health. Your body also releases hormones during sleep that help repair daily wear and

HISTORICAL SLEEP ACCOMMODATIONS

Sleep has always been a valued commodity, which shows in how beds were built through time. Ancient Chinese beds looked like little houses placed in the middle of the room. Ancient Egyptians constructed wooden beds sloped up toward the head. Ancient Greeks used couches for reclining during the day that doubled as beds at night — and decorated them elaborately. Ancient Romans too used ornate couches embellished with bronze, silver and gold.

tear in your cells and affect how your body burns energy.

Recent research suggests that the brain does its "chores" during shut-eye. While you sleep, your brain flushes toxins and other byproducts out of its cellular metabolism. Moreover, it seems that the deeper the sleep, the better the cleaning system works.

You may think that lack of sleep is fixable with coffee and other caffeinated drinks, but while they keep you awake, they don't provide the restorative function of slumber. Without enough sleep, your brain can't perform its housekeeping tasks, leaving you struggling to focus, process information and remember things. This can lead to loss of productivity, injuries and accidents — even tragic ones. And ongoing sleep deprivation impacts your long-term health, contributing to chronic conditions such as heart disease, stroke, high blood pressure, diabetes, kidney and liver disease, and depression.

WHAT IS SLEEP HYGIENE?

Sleep experts often toss around the term *sleep hygiene*. They use it to describe your approach toward your sleep habits as well as your daily and nightly routine, behaviors and environment.

Tips for better sleep

Sleep is therapeutic and it's available for free, without a prescription — it's one of the best holistic therapies you can have. Like any medicine, sleep must be taken regularly. To make the most of your nightly dose of sleep, consider the following tips.

Make sleep a priority

It may be tempting to stay up late studying, working or scrolling through social media and then rush to get to sleep. But respecting your need for sleep is key to holistic well-being. Going through a bedtime ritual signals your mind and body that sleep is imminent. Focus on bedtime habits that relax you and allow you to release the day's stressors. These might include taking a bath, getting into comfortable pajamas, meditating or reading. The activity itself isn't as important as its calming effects.

Stick to a sleep schedule

Go to bed and get up at the same time every day, including weekends. Being consistent reinforces your body's sleep-wake cycle. Children and adults sleep better when they have a bedtime routine. Stick to a regular sleep routine. Doing the same thing before bed each night can help prepare your body for rest and condition your brain for sleep.

SLEEP AIDS

Taking medication to help you sleep can be tempting. If you have a short-term sleep issue, such as jet lag or a period of high stress, a prescription sleeping pill may be helpful. Keep in mind that sleeping pills have side effects and over the long term can cause dependence and other problems while not helping you get better-quality sleep.

If you regularly have trouble getting to sleep or staying asleep, commonly known as insomnia, talk to your primary care team or a sleep specialist. The best way to manage insomnia often depends on what's causing it. Identifying and managing an underlying disorder, such as anxiety or sleep apnea, is much more effective than just treating the symptom of insomnia.

Create a restful environment
Make your room conducive to sleep by keeping it cool, dark and quiet. Consider using room-darkening shades, earplugs, a fan or other devices to create an environment that suits your needs. Smartphone apps that produce white noise can help mask unwanted sounds.

Shut off devices
Avoid prolonged use of light-emitting screens just before bedtime. The artificial light suppresses the body's natural production of melatonin. So even when we finally turn off the lights and devices, our stimulated brains can't instantly settle into the state of slumber, making it harder to fall asleep and contributing to insomnia.

Manage stress
How you handle stress can significantly affect your ability to fall and stay asleep. If your busy mind keeps you up at night, give yourself the opportunity to quiet your thoughts. Jot down what's on your mind and then set it aside for tomorrow. Meditation, aromatherapy, deep breathing or keeping a gratitude journal also may help invite quality sleep. (Learn more about aromatherapy, deep breathing and meditation on pages 80, 109 and 148.)

Include physical activity in your daily routine
Regular physical activity during the day can promote better sleep at night. Just avoid being active too close to bedtime. Spending time outside every day might be helpful too.

Keep naps short
Long daytime naps can interfere with nighttime sleep. Limit naps to no more than one hour and avoid napping late in the day. If you work nights, however, you might need to nap late in the day before work to help make up for any sleep deficiencies.

Limit foods and drinks before bed
Don't go to bed on a full stomach (or a hungry one). In particular, avoid heavy or large meals within a couple of hours of bedtime because digestive discomfort can keep you up. Nicotine, caffeine and alcohol deserve caution too. The stimulating effects of nicotine and caffeine take hours to wear off and can interfere with sleep. And even though alcohol might make you feel sleepy at first, it can disrupt sleep later in the night. To avoid multiple bathroom trips during the night, limit your water intake before bedtime. If you have an overactive bladder, minimizing acidic foods before bedtime can help.

Get out of bed
Do you toss and turn and just can't fall asleep? It may be time to get up for a bit. If you lie in bed stressing about your inability to doze off, get out of bed and do something that promotes relaxation. This might be reading, practicing guided imagery (page 113) or focusing on your breath (page 109). When you begin to feel sleepy, head back to bed. Limit spending time in bed frustrated about not being able to fall asleep.

NUTRITION
What you eat has a direct effect on how you feel and how your body functions. A healthy diet — one that emphasizes vegetables, fruits, lean proteins and whole grains — may lower your risk of diseases.

Whole, minimally processed foods offer much more value in terms of health benefits than do ultraprocessed foods.

Ultraprocessed foods are manufactured for convenience and taste, and are usually high in sugar, fat, sodium and preservatives. A few examples are soft drinks; prepackaged meals, cookies and snacks; ready mixes; and candies. Because these foods are typically low in fiber, people often need to eat a greater volume of them compared with whole foods to feel full. On the other hand, a diet of primarily whole foods is low in calories and rich in nutrients.

What to eat
To eat healthy, it may not be necessary to follow a special diet. The goal is to eat a variety of healthy foods that taste good and are good for you.

Vegetables and fruits

Every day, researchers learn more and more about how vegetables and fruits supply the body with a variety of substances to ward off illness. These bright and colorful foods are loaded with health-promoting vitamins, minerals and fiber. Fiber reduces inflammation and improves the diversity of the gut microbiome — the healthy, beneficial bacteria living in your body.

In addition to their anti-inflammatory properties, vegetables and fruits have antioxidant, anticancer and antiviral effects. People who typically eat generous helpings of vegetables and fruits are at lower risk of developing many ailments that are leading causes of death, including:

- Heart disease
- High blood pressure
- Cancer
- Diabetes

Carbohydrates

When it comes to carbohydrates, the key word to remember is *whole*, as in *whole grains* (not to be confused with *multigrain*). The less refined a carbohydrate food is, the better it is for your health. Unrefined whole grains abound in fiber, vitamins, minerals and other important nutrients.

Choose whole-grain breads, pastas and cereals whenever you can, and experiment with whole grains such as farro or bulgur. Save the other end of the spectrum — ultraprocessed foods with refined sugar, such as cookies, candies and soft drinks — for special occasions.

Protein and dairy

It's not necessary to eat meat every day. Although meat is rich in protein, many cuts of meat are high in saturated fat and cholesterol. When you do eat meat, choose lean cuts.

What's on your plate is one important
aspect of good nutrition. But *how* you eat
is another key to healthy eating. Take time
to savor and enjoy the experience.

A variety of other foods furnish protein too, including:
- Dairy products, such as yogurt.
- Seafood.
- Legumes, such as beans, lentils and peas.

These foods provide other benefits as well. For example, dairy products are rich in calcium and vitamin D, and seafood often supplies omega-3 fatty acids, which are heart- and brain-healthy. Try to substitute these foods for meat regularly.

Fats

Some fats are good for you. Nuts, for instance, contain fat but also vitamin E, which can be beneficial for eye health. Research shows that people who replace much of the animal fat in their meals with plant-based oils, such as olive or canola oil, can reduce their blood cholesterol level. While nuts and plant-based oils may have health benefits, keep in mind they are high in calories, so moderation is key.

Sweets

Sweets are high in calories and offer little nutrition. That doesn't mean they're not nice to have on occasion. You don't have to give up sweets entirely to eat well, but be smart about your selections and portion sizes. Small portions of chocolate — especially dark chocolate — contain antioxidants that even provide some health benefits.

Alcohol

Like sweets, alcohol is high in calories and low in healthy nutrients. In the past, a glass of red wine a day was thought to be part of a healthy diet, but more recent studies have found few health benefits related to alcohol.

Drinking any amount of alcohol is associated with health risks. Certainly, it can cause intoxication. Alcohol also impairs brain function, perhaps even long term, negatively impacts sleep quality, can lead to indigestion, and contributes to health problems such as addiction, liver disease and certain cancers. If you already drink at low levels and continue to drink, risks for these issues appear to be low. But the risk is not zero. Avoid all alcohol if you:
- Are trying to get pregnant or are pregnant.
- Take medicine that has side effects that are worse with alcohol.
- Have alcohol use disorder.
- Have medical issues that alcohol can worsen.

If you drink socially or as a way to relax, consider less-risky alternatives such as sipping nonalcoholic drinks, doing yoga or just being outside.

How you eat

What's on your plate is one important aspect of good nutrition. But *how* you eat is another key to healthy eating. Consider these questions:

- Do you eat while doing something else, such as watching television, reading a book or using a computer or other electronic device?
- Do you eat while you're at your desk in the office or in the car on the way to work?

IT'S THE PATTERN THAT MATTERS

It's not always easy to tease out specific associations between health benefits and certain foods. What research has found, more often than not, is that certain patterns of eating tend to be associated with better health. For example, plant-based diets along with lean proteins have the greatest benefit in preventing chronic conditions such as heart disease, cancer and dementia.

The Mediterranean diet, which is plant-focused, is one such diet. The Mayo Clinic diet, which is similar in many ways to the Mediterranean diet, is another. So is the Dietary Approaches to Stop Hypertension (DASH) diet, which places more emphasis on lowering sodium intake, as well as the MIND (Mediterranean-DASH Intervention for Neurodegenerative Delay) diet, which focuses on brain health.

An important benefit of these plant-based eating plans is their anti-inflammatory effect — the way they help reduce chronic low-grade inflammation, a mechanism that underlies so many chronic diseases.

The fruits, vegetables and whole grains found in these diets increase consumption of soluble fiber, which is important for its anti-inflammatory properties. Healthy sources of fat, such as olive oil, increase intake of monounsaturated fats, which are also anti-inflammatory. Fish, another staple of these diets, is rich in omega-3 fatty acids, a type of polyunsaturated fat also thought to curb inflammation.

The anti-inflammatory properties of these dietary approaches appear to directly correlate with why they decrease the risk of death from heart disease, stroke and cancer, as well as lower the risk of developing diabetes, Alzheimer's disease, arthritis, Parkinson's disease and other illnesses.

- How much attention do you pay to what you're eating?
- At what pace do you tend to eat? Do you eat slowly, or do you eat quickly?

Depending on how you answered these questions, practicing mindfulness at your next meal may be another way that you can improve your approach to eating.

Mindfulness, in a traditional sense, means being present in the moment (see page 148). Eating mindfully means taking time to eat and be fully aware of the tastes and textures of the food in your mouth. By doing this, you slow down, giving your body a chance to experience the food and tell you when you've had enough. Other ways to slow down and notice your meals include putting your fork down or taking sips of water between bites.

Getting into a healthy groove
With everything that you have to do each day, making sure that you and your family eat healthy meals may seem difficult and time-consuming.

When it comes to cooking, many people feel that they don't have the time. That's because healthy eating is often associated with complicated recipes, time-intensive meal preparation and added trips to the grocery store. However, you can prepare a healthy meal as quickly as you can prepare an unhealthy one. Here are several ways you can eat well without a lot of fuss and hassle.

Plan by the week
It can be more efficient to plan meals for an entire week, especially if you shop for groceries on a weekly basis. Planning your meals each week allows you time to choose healthy meals. It will also help ensure that you have all of the right ingredients on hand when it's time to prepare breakfast, lunch or dinner.

Look for shortcuts
Another way to simplify meal preparation and save time is to purchase precut vegetables and fruits, precooked meats and packaged salads. Frozen vegetables are a cost-effective option that keep longer than fresh produce and may come in handy for some dishes.

Shop from a list
Following a list helps you stick to your meal plan and keeps you from impulse buying. This helps your health and your budget. Try to avoid shopping when you're hungry — you may be tempted to grab anything that looks appetizing.

EASY WAYS TO EAT MEDITERRANEAN

Research shows that people who follow the traditional Mediterranean way of eating tend to have good heart health. Here are some tips if you want to follow suit:

- **Eat more fruits and vegetables** Eat fruit for breakfast. Fill half your dinner plate with vegetables.
- **Choose whole grains** Switch to whole-grain bread, cereal and pasta. You also can try other whole grains, such as bulgur, barley and farro.
- **Use plant-based oils** Olive oil is the big one, of course, but you also can experiment with safflower, grapeseed and avocado oils.
- **Eat more seafood** Eat fish or shellfish 2 or 3 times a week. Fresh or water-packed tuna, salmon, trout, mackerel and herring are healthy choices.
- **Get nuts** Have a handful of raw, unsalted nuts as a snack a few times a week.
- **Enjoy some dairy** Some good choices are skim or low-fat milk, cottage cheese, and Greek or plain yogurt.
- **Reduce red and processed meat** Eat more fish, poultry or beans instead. If you eat meat, make sure it's lean and keep portions small.
- **Spice it up** Herbs and spices boost flavor and lessen the need for salt.

Adapt to the seasons
Whenever you can, look for recently harvested produce. Here are some examples:
- **Spring:** asparagus, peas, cherries
- **Midsummer:** peaches, sweet corn, tomatoes
- **Fall:** apples, pears, squash

Depending on the season and where you live, look for farmers markets near you. Farmers markets offer local produce, which tends to be the freshest around.

Be adventurous
Discovering new foods and flavors is part of the joy of cooking and eating, so don't be afraid to explore unfamiliar cuisines. Keep in mind that the

broadest range of health benefits comes from meals that feature a wide variety of foods.

Be flexible
Remember that every food you eat doesn't have to be an excellent source of nutrients. Nor is it out of the question to eat high-fat, high-calorie foods on occasion. The main thing is that you choose foods that promote good health more often than you choose those that don't.

STRESS MANAGEMENT
Modern life is filled with stress. According to a recent survey by the American Psychological Association, the most common stressors range from fears of mass shootings and worries about the economy to concerns about healthcare, work-related pressures and money. The COVID-19 pandemic, global conflicts, racial injustice, inflation and climate-related disasters add to the sources of stress.

Stress is a natural human response that evolved to address threats and ensure survival. Early humans developed the so-called fight-or-flight stress response to help them fight off predators or escape them. This stress response still works the same way today. When encountering a perceived threat — be it a dangerous driving situation, a conflict at work or worry about being late — the body activates the same biological gears.

The body's stress response
First, a part of the brain called the hypothalamus detects the threat. Then it sends a message to the adrenal glands, located atop the kidneys.

The adrenal glands release a surge of hormones, including adrenaline and cortisol. Adrenaline increases heart rate, elevates blood pressure and boosts energy. Cortisol, the primary stress hormone, drives up glucose in the bloodstream, enhances the brain's use of glucose and increases the availability of substances that repair tissues. Cortisol also dampens functions that aren't useful for a fight-or-flight response, such as activities of the immune and digestive systems. Once the perceived threat is gone, the adrenaline and cortisol levels drop and your body's processes return to normal.

This quick succession of physiological events enabled early humans to run fast or fight back efficiently. While it's still useful today, most modern humans encounter far fewer life-threatening events on a regular basis.

The problem of modern stress
Running away from a hungry bear is a good use of the fight-or-flight response. Thinking about running away from a bear is not, although the

34   Mayo Clinic Guide to Holistic Health

STRESS MANAGEMENT TIPS

Stephen Kopecky, M.D., a cardiologist at Mayo Clinic, offers these tips for de-stressing:

- **Practice positive self talk** The goal of positive self-talk is to weed out misconceptions and challenge them with self-compassion and rational, positive thoughts. Start by following one simple rule: Don't say anything to yourself that you wouldn't say to a friend or loved one. Be gentle and encouraging with yourself. If a negative thought enters your mind, evaluate it rationally and respond with affirmations of what is good about you.
- **Indulge your senses** A simple way to de-stress is to engage your senses — touch, smell, sight, taste and hearing. "To deal with work stress," Dr. Kopecky says, "I started to use aromatherapy in the office (smell), brought in a beautiful oriental rug (sight) with a thick cushion pad underneath it to make it more comfortable to stand on (touch), and subscribed to a music service that provided relaxing classical music (hearing). These changes, while small, have helped me tremendously to manage my stress throughout the day, and I have noticed colleagues doing the same. Some even come into my office and say, 'Can I just sit here for a few moments to relax?' to which my response is 'Please — be my guest.'"
- **Get outside** Studies show that spending time in nature reduces stress, lowers cortisol levels, decreases blood pressure and improves well-being. As little as 10 minutes in a green space can make a significant difference in your mood and stress level, whether you're taking a stroll or sitting down and enjoying the view. If you want to experience an even greater drop in stress, try spending 20 to 30 minutes at a time in a natural setting. For many of us the sounds, sights and smells of green spaces — such as forests, wetlands, city parks and gardens — have a powerful calming effect. (Read more about forest bathing on page 47.)

act of thinking about something stressful can trigger almost the same physiological response as physically reacting to the stressor.

Say you're stuck in traffic and feel stressed about it. Your endocrine system will likely release adrenaline and cortisol, as it's programmed to

Whole-health fundamentals **35**

do, but there's nothing for which you can use that response — you can't fight the car in front of you and you can't run away because you're stuck in your car. Human stressors have switched from bears to traffic jams in just a couple of generations. But our basic hardwired system hasn't changed. This means we are all leaking a lot of adrenaline and cortisol every day. When stress hormones flood the body but aren't used, they contribute to low-level inflammation throughout the body, reduced immunity and other health problems.

The problem is twofold: On the one hand, our bodies are using an old system to deal with new problems, such as meeting increasing demands for productivity and keeping up with a nonstop digital world. On the other hand, this system gets triggered multiple times a day. Eventually, the negative effects of a continuously activated stress response system accumulate.

Chronic activation of the stress-response system can disrupt almost all body processes. This can cause health problems that impact quality of life and increase the chances of disease and early death. Chronic stress can cause:

- **Heart disease** Stress raises your heart rate and increases inflammation, including in the arteries that supply blood to your heart.
- **Diabetes** Living with high levels of stress hormones can interfere with your body's ability to use insulin efficiently. This can lead to developing or worsening type 2 diabetes.
- **Weight gain** The body's stress response system is linked to regulation of appetite and energy. High stress can prompt you to eat more than you intended, which can lead to weight gain. Chronic stress also may stimulate metabolic processes that promote storage of fat.
- **Poor brain health** Stress can impact your ability to think, learn and store memories. Research suggests that stress may increase the risk of certain forms of dementia, including Alzheimer's.
- **Weakened immune system** Stress hormones may disrupt or suppress your immune system so that it has a harder time fighting infection.

React to stress in a healthy way

While it's unlikely you'll be able to eliminate stress from your life, you can learn ways to minimize its effects. Many of the therapies detailed in the "Therapies A–Z" section, such as yoga, deep breathing, massage and meditation, work to help decrease stress. You can also aim for at least 30 minutes a day of one of these activities:

- Take care of the basics. Eat a healthy diet (see page 28) and get regular exercise (see page 21). Get plenty of sleep too (see page 25).
- Keep a journal. Write about your thoughts or what you're grateful for in your life.

36   Mayo Clinic Guide to Holistic Health

PREJUDICES AND PRINCIPLES

In his book *The Mayo Clinic Guide to Stress-Free Living*, Amit Sood, M.D., explains how prejudices cause stress and how principles can lead to stress-free living.

Prejudices are overgeneralized, self-focused shortcuts that create a rigid, often negative worldview. They originate in the mind's survival instinct. Prejudices see the world in black and white — good or bad, like it or hate it — despite the fact that most things are gray. Prejudices strain relationships and can lead to conflicts. Much of the world's unrest originates from prejudices.

Principles originate in the wisdom gained from deeper reflections. They teach you to accept the gray areas, embracing life's uncertainties. With training, introspection and time, prejudices can give way to principles, helping build a more flexible view of the world. Here are five healthy principles to live by.

- **Gratitude** acknowledges your blessings, little or large. Clean air, drinkable water, nourishing food, safety, love, respect and the opportunity to pursue excellence are all immeasurably valuable gifts. Don't wait until you lose your gifts to appreciate their value.
- **Compassion** recognizes and honors the pain and suffering of all life forms and intends to heal with words and actions.
- **Acceptance** embraces life's uncertainties by letting go of the uncontrollable and engaging with the present. You find moments each day to pause and appreciate the flowers that have bloomed in your life's garden.
- **Higher meaning** focuses on who you are, why you are here and what this world means. You touch a part of the world, however small, and leave it a little better and happier than you found it.
- **Forgiveness** respects each person's humanness, recognizing we all are fallible and vulnerable to ignorant thoughts and actions. Forgiveness is your gift to yourself and others — a gift that provides peace and freedom to all.

- Take time for hobbies, such as honing a craft or listening to music.
- Foster healthy friendships and talk with friends and family (see next section).
- Find ways to include humor and laughter in your life, such as watching funny movies or learning a good joke you can retell.

Whole-health fundamentals

- Volunteer in your community.
- Get organized. Focus on what you need to get done at home and work. Remove tasks that aren't needed.

SOCIAL CONNECTEDNESS

In March 2020, when countries across the globe went into lockdown to prevent the spread of COVID-19, one of the factors that affected people most was the abrupt disconnect from the social life they had been accustomed to.

Working adults missed their office colleagues. Grandparents missed their grandchildren. Teenagers missed hanging out at their friends' houses. Young parents missed socializing together while their children played or napped in strollers. Friends missed spending weekends together. Older adults missed meeting at libraries, in coffee shops or for walks.

If there was one thing that the global pandemic clearly revealed, it was the importance of social connections.

Social connectedness is the degree to which people have and perceive relationships. This includes the desired number, quality and diversity of relationships and how they create feelings of belonging, worth and support. When we lost the ability to see each other in person, our sense of connectedness suffered. Even with virtual interactions, many people still felt lonely.

Loneliness is the opposite of connectedness. Loneliness reflects the difference between a person's actual and desired level of connection. Not having meaningful or close relationships or a sense of belonging can produce feelings of loneliness.

Prolonged loneliness often leads to emotional distress, depression and anxiety. Left untended, loneliness may have serious consequences for memory, emotions, behavior and health. Chronic loneliness and social isolation can increase the risk of dementia by approximately 50%.

According to surveys, more than 1 in 3 adults age 45 and older feel lonely in the United States. Overall, scientists calculate that lacking social connectedness is as dangerous as smoking 15 cigarettes a day.

Humans are social beings — they need to be around each other. Warm family ties and good friendships contribute to mental and emotional well-being throughout life. Family and friends keep you grounded and provide love and support through life's ups and downs.

But friendship is good for you in more ways than you may realize. Studies also show that people who enjoy strong, healthy connections with family, friends and partners tend to have better physical health as well as increased longevity.

WHAT IF YOU'RE AN INTROVERT?

For some people, the prospect of spending a lot of time with others can seem more stressful than energizing. What if you're the type of person who recharges their social battery by being alone rather than spending time with people? That's perfectly OK too. Don't feel that you must force social interaction if you don't want it or need it.

Being alone is not the same thing as being lonely (see page 38). Some people meet their needs for connectedness through pets, nature or spiritual activities that give them many of the same benefits as human interactions. For an introvert, being alone can be a form of self-care. The point is not that you're physically surrounded by people, but that you feel supported and that you're comfortable where you are in the world.

Benefits of relationships

Research indicates that physical health is substantially affected by the quantity and quality of your social relationships. An analysis of combined data from four long-term studies among age groups ranging from adolescence through late adulthood suggests that at each phase in life, social connectedness is an important predictor of future physical health.

The analysis showed that strong social support and low social strain were linked to positive effects on biological health markers. In particular, strong social support in late adulthood was linked to lower blood pressure and body mass index (BMI). Low social strain, indicated by lack of tension and conflict in relationships, was associated with lower waist circumference and BMI, as well as lower levels of chronic inflammation in mid- to late adulthood.

A study following more than 7,500 Australian women over 20 years found that those having satisfying social connections had fewer chronic illnesses than those who reported lower relationship satisfaction.

Studies also show a clear link between social relationships and longevity. Across the globe, loneliness is associated with an earlier death. When various facets of social connectedness are measured, a rich social life tends to increase the odds of survival substantially, especially in young and middle-aged adults. Protective effects appear to rival those of other health-promoting lifestyle factors such as healthy weight, physical activity, smoking cessation and flu vaccinations.

Researchers following a large group of socioeconomically diverse African American men and women with a broad age range came to similar conclusions. They found that a higher level of social integration — being married or living together, having six or more close friends or relatives, attending weekly religious services and belonging to four or more social or church groups — was strongly associated with a lower risk of premature death.

THE POWER OF A POSITIVE OUTLOOK

Is your glass half empty or half full? How you answer this timeless question may reflect your outlook on life, your attitude toward yourself and those around you, and your overall quality of life. Research suggests that optimism and pessimism are more than just character traits. The way you see that glass may affect your health, well-being and even life span, studies find.

A recent study examined up to 26 years of data shared by thousands of postmenopausal women. The researchers found that women who were more optimistic lived about four years longer than those who scored lower on optimism assessments. Even after adjusting for medical history, education and income, the connection between optimism and longevity was still strong.

Another recent study examined the links between optimism, stress and emotional well-being in older men. Investigators found that men who were more optimistic experienced fewer negative emotions. Researchers pinned that connection on fewer daily stressors, positing that optimism may help older adults avoid, pivot away from or change how they think about stressful moments.

For many people, stress is a daily occurrence. It's just not possible to eliminate it completely. However, it is possible to reduce its ill effects. Optimism is a tendency to expect good things in the future. Optimists do that well, and they also tend to be confident and persistent when faced with difficulties. They expect good outcomes, even when things are hard, which results in a relatively positive mix of emotions.

Even if you aren't naturally inclined to optimism, you can learn to be more positive. The process of turning a negative outlook into a positive one is simple, but it takes time and practice. Essentially, you're creating a new habit. Here are some ways to think and behave in a more positive and optimistic way:

40 Mayo Clinic Guide to Holistic Health

Finding the link

Researchers suspect that being connected with others protects your physical health by:

- Enabling you to get better or more prompt medical care, or actually providing you with medical care.
- Motivating you to engage in healthy behaviors, such as walking regularly or quitting smoking.

- **Identify areas to change** First identify areas of your life that you usually think negatively about, whether it's work, your daily commute, life changes or a relationship. You can start small by focusing on one area to approach in a more positive manner. Think of constructive ways to manage your stress instead of counterproductive ones.
- **Check yourself** Periodically during the day, stop and evaluate what you're thinking. If you find that your thoughts are mainly pessimistic, try to find a way to put a hopeful spin on them.
- **Be open to humor** Give yourself permission to smile or laugh, especially during difficult times. Seek humor in everyday happenings. When you can laugh at life, you feel less stressed.
- **Follow a healthy lifestyle** Aim to exercise for about 30 minutes most days of the week. You also can break it up into 5- or 10-minute chunks of time during the day. Exercise can positively affect mood and reduce stress. Follow a healthy diet to fuel your mind and body. Get enough sleep. And learn techniques to manage stress.
- **Surround yourself with positive people** Make sure those in your life are positive, supportive people you can depend on to give helpful advice and feedback. Negative people may increase your stress level and make you doubt your ability to manage stress in healthy ways.
- **Practice self-compassion** Dr. Sood (see page 37) links self-compassion to being kind and comforting to yourself while accepting your imperfections and acknowledging your place in the wider world. He explains that being compassionate to yourself doesn't make you self-indulgent or narcissistic. On the contrary, accepting yourself motivates you to accept others.

- Providing you with practical help when needed — for example, assistance with household chores and transportation.
- Reducing stress and anxiety, which can have negative health consequences.
- Allowing you to receive direct expressions of affection, esteem and respect (socioemotional support), which in turn might increase your biological resistance to disease.
- Allowing you to give support and perform well in the role of friend or family member, increasing your sense of purpose and mastery of life.
- Altering physiological pathways, such as boosting your immune system and moderating hormone and cardiovascular reactivity.

Building quality relationships

During a person's busy midlife years, working and raising children often take priority over other things, including friendships and maybe even spousal or family relationships. You may have grown apart due to changes in your lives or interests. Or maybe you've moved to a new community and haven't yet found a way to meet people.

Developing and maintaining good relationships takes effort, but the multiple benefits are worth it. Even as adults, it's important to remember that to have good friends, it's important to be a good friend, even to people in your own family. Good friends:

- Like, respect and trust each other.
- Accept each other even though they don't always understand each other.
- Allow space for each other to grow, change and make decisions, even if there's disagreement.
- Listen and share freely, without judging or criticizing.
- Respect each other's boundaries.
- Don't take advantage of each other.
- Accept and give help as needed.
- Don't reveal private information about each other to others.
- Have each other's best interests in mind.
- Are there for each other but are not obsessed with each other.
- Have individual as well as mutual interests.

Friends don't always come in the same shapes and sizes. Be open to people outside your immediate demographic — you might be surprised at what someone who's younger or from a different racial, ethnic or religious background can bring to the table. Also, keep in mind that there are different levels of friendship. Some are very close, others more superficial, but all can be beneficial.

SPIRITUALITY AND PURPOSE

Does health have a spiritual dimension? The spiritual aspect of life can be difficult to observe in medical studies. But it's equally difficult to dismiss the power of transcendent experiences.

Spirituality is paradoxically ubiquitous and elusive, as it can mean something different to each person. In general, it encompasses our search for meaning and purpose in life as well as the connections we make with others. It also includes how we view our inner selves and our surroundings. As a result, how it is felt and practiced is highly personal.

For some, spirituality is closely tied to religious beliefs and activities, such as prayer and participation in a religious community. For others, it's being in nature and honoring that; yet others find spirituality in music and art. And some individuals view spirituality as simply experiencing a sense of peace, purpose or connection to others. Notably, spirituality doesn't create silos. It transcends barriers because it allows us to see ourselves in others. Accepting others is profoundly spiritual.

"Spirituality is not constrained to religious practices," says this book's editor, Brent A. Bauer, M.D., director of research for the Mayo Clinic Integrative Medicine and Health program. "Spirituality is what brings meaning to your life. And it's about honoring the things that are important to you."

Spirituality is sometimes referred to as inner strength. It plays an important role in how we cope with illness, grief and anxiety, and how we achieve healing and a sense of coherence. Positive spiritual experiences can bring a sense of oneness and connection to others, to a higher power, or to the natural world. Spirituality can provide a pathway for forgiveness, gratitude and joy, and be restorative, rejuvenating and healing.

Benefits of spirituality

Modern medicine has typically viewed itself as grounded firmly in science and separate from religious or spiritual matters. But matters such as religion and spirituality are important and growing evidence suggests that religion and spirituality can have a measurable impact on health. More recently, researchers have been examining how spirituality can support health in the contexts of medicine, nursing, ethics, social work and psychology.

Spirituality appears to have benefits for stress relief and overall mental health. It can help you:

- **Feel a sense of purpose** Cultivating your spirituality may help uncover what's most meaningful to you. Knowing where to invest your energy and resources can motivate you to live intentionally, cope with ongoing stress and take better care of yourself and your health.
- **Feel more connected** The more you feel you have a purpose in the world, the less solitary you may feel — even when you're alone. This

Whole-health fundamentals **43**

feeling of connectedness can lead to fewer depressive symptoms and improved mental health.

- **Release control** When you feel part of a greater whole, you may realize that you aren't responsible for everything that happens in life. You can share the burden of tough times as well as the joys of life's blessings with those around you. Releasing control can help you better manage stress.
- **Expand your support network** Whether you find spirituality in a place of worship, in your family or in nature walks with a friend, this sharing of spiritual expression can help build relationships.

Cultivating your spirituality

Even if you don't necessarily think of yourself as a very spiritual person, there likely are certain things that move you deeply. Humans have an inborn capacity to experience transcendence — a spiritual state, or a condition of moving beyond physical needs and realities.

Cultivating a deeper spirituality means getting in touch with your inner self as well as embodying love, expressed as gratitude, compassion, acceptance, forgiveness, hope and unselfishness.

- Try prayer, meditation or mindfulness to help focus your thoughts and to find peace.
- Keep a journal to help you express your feelings and record progress.
- Find a trusted adviser or friend who can help you discover what's important to you in life. Others may have insights that you haven't yet discovered.
- Read inspirational stories or essays to help you evaluate different philosophies of life.
- Talk to others whose spiritual lives you admire. Ask questions to learn how they found their way to a fulfilling spiritual life.

You also can explore your spirituality by thinking about:

- Your important relationships.
- What you value most in your life.
- The people who give you a sense of community.
- What inspires you and gives you hope.
- What brings you joy.
- Your proudest achievements.

Exploring these ideas can help you find a sense of purpose and meaning within yourself and in your relationships with others. Knowing what matters can offer hope and peace during times of struggle or personal crisis. Following your guiding principles can lead to positive changes and improve your quality of life.

Following your guiding principles can lead to positive changes and improve your quality of life.

Looking outside yourself

Spirituality is also nurtured by your relationships with others. Fostering relationships with the people who are important to you can lead to a deepened sense of your place in life and in the greater good. To do this:

- Make relationships with friends and family a priority. Give more than you receive.
- See the good in people and in yourself. Accept others as they are, without judgment.
- Contribute to your community by being neighborly, volunteering and participating in civic groups.

Spirituality and health

Addressing spiritual needs is an important aspect of holistic health. Having a sense of purpose and connection to something outside yourself often accompanies other whole-health promoters, such as gratitude, compassion, mindfulness, and prayer or meditation.

In the context of a medical illness, spirituality becomes a source of strength, enabling people to persevere rather than feeling overpowered by the disease. It can be a comfort in times of profound suffering, such as losing a loved one, being diagnosed with a terminal disease or witnessing a natural disaster. People who experience a severe trauma or a life-threatening illness often describe a renewed sense of appreciation for life, which can be spiritual.

Overall, spirituality can provide social support, decrease stress, improve mood and foster a healthy relationship with the body. It's a tool every human comes equipped with, and it's yours to explore and develop.

CONNECTION WITH NATURE

Have you ever noticed that walking in a forest puts you in a better mood? Or that strolling on the beach or watching a sunset fills you with peace and joy? Does listening to birds sing or watching butterflies flutter around flowers instill within you a sense of wonder? If so, you're not alone. Other people experience similar positive outcomes when they spend a day or even a few hours in nature. There's a reason for it. We evolved with nature around us — first as hunter-gatherers who roamed the earth, and then as farmers who spent much of their time in the fields.

This deep-seated need to connect with the natural world, also called biophilia, is universal among humans. American biologist Edward O. Wilson proposed in the mid-1980s that humans have an innate connection with the natural world and a desire to engage with other forms of life, be it plants and trees or birds and animals. That's why we feel so refreshed after spending time outdoors. We quench our innate cravings for nature.

More than half the people on the planet today live in cities, and by 2050, this number is expected to hit 70%. Urban life offers many advantages — career choices, social interactions, restaurants, entertainment and nightlife. Yet, despite all that, urbanization is associated with increased levels of mental illness, and it isn't entirely clear why.

Many urban dwellers spend most of their lives inside offices and apartments — in the global North, humans stay inside approximately 90% of the time. With such living arrangements, we are missing nature's restorative effects on our physical and mental health, researchers say. After all, on the evolutionary scale, city living is a fairly recent development. For most of human history, we spent far more time in nature's embrace than we do now.

Nature effects
Exactly how does nature affect us? Scientists are working to measure and quantify its effects on our mind and body.

Mind
Nature has tangible mental effects. One study, for example, found that nature walks reduce rumination — a repetitive thinking or dwelling on negative feelings, emotions, causes and consequences — which can spiral into anxiety or depression. Researchers observed that a 90-minute nature walk quieted neural activity in the prefrontal cortex, the part of the brain that regulates thoughts, actions and emotions. A similar walk taken in urban settings did not have the same healthy outcome. However, walking through a city park had comparable positive effects, as noted in another study that focused specifically on urban green spaces.

Scientists now understand the neural underpinnings of this phenomenon better. As we admire flowers, watch birds fly or listen to a waterfall splash, our minds enter the so-called state of soft fascination. What happens is this: Initially, the mind is drawn to the fascinating aspects of nature. Then it wanders in various directions. This allows new thoughts or ideas to arise — and possibly even stimulates creativity.

> Shinrin-yoku ("forest bathing") — the practice of spending sensory-focused time in a forest or other natural environment — lowers blood pressure, heart rate and stress hormones.

As the brain rests, its ability to focus is renewed, restoring attention. Hard fascination, in which our attention is strongly captured — such as when we are watching TV or working — doesn't produce the same restorative effect.

Body
Nature also has physiological effects. In 1982, the Japanese Ministry of Agriculture, Forestry and Fisheries coined the term *shinrin-yoku*, which translates to "forest bathing." Studies have found that forest bathing — spending sensory-focused time in a forest or other natural environment — lowers blood pressure, heart rate and stress hormones.

A large study that followed over 100,000 women found that being surrounded with greenery extends life span. Another research effort revealed that greater exposure to green vegetation boosts survival chances after stroke in men and women. Having a hospital window with a view has been shown to improve healing and recovery after surgery, with fewer complications and less pain medication needed.

Nature prescriptions
Don't be surprised if at your next medical appointment you get a prescription not for pills but for parks. More and more healthcare professionals are including nature therapy in their recommendations. Moreover, it seems that nature's healing touch can sometimes be nothing short of amazing.

Jean Larson, assistant professor of nature-based therapeutics at the Bakken Center and director of nature-based therapy services at the Minnesota Landscape Arboretum, recently observed that being in nature improves symptoms in people with Parkinson's disease. When patients are engaged with nature activities, their Parkinson's symptoms improve, she found. "The brain is distracted," she says. "And instead of perseverating on what they can't do, they are engaged in what they are doing and concentrating on that instead of their tremors."

Park Rx America is a nonprofit organization dedicated to increasing awareness of nature's health benefits for everyone. You can learn more on their website, *www.parkrxamerica.org*, and even write your own nature prescription.

Biophilic indoor spaces

Being able to regularly enjoy nature is great, but what if you live in a city, far from a park, and don't have a garden? Don't despair. Having some biophilic elements in your home or workplace also can have restorative effects.

To investigate how biophilic environments impact people, Mayo Clinic researchers set up special immersion rooms that included various nature-mimicking elements. One type of room was furnished with various indoor plants and images of tall, canopy-type trees and shrubs were projected onto the walls. In another, speakers played natural sounds such as wind blowing through trees, gentle trickles of streams, chirping crickets and the calls of birds native to the American Midwest. Finally, the third type of setup included both the visual and the auditory elements.

Throughout their workday, study participants wore trackers on their wrists that measured their physiological indicators of stress, such as changes in heart rate and sweat, which the scientists recorded.

The study found that, overall, biophilic indoor settings helped reduce work-related stress, improve cognitive performance and increase participants' overall satisfaction with their environments. The combination of visual and auditory elements provided the most benefits.

AMBIENT THERAPY

Chip Davis, composer and founder of Mannheim Steamroller, is probably best known for his Christmas music. But he's also teamed up with experts at Mayo Clinic and other health institutions to bring a new experience to patients called ambient therapy. Davis created a customized recording system to capture three-dimensional nature sounds. These sounds were then piped into operating rooms and patient rooms at Mayo Clinic. The goal was to make patients feel as if they'd been transported to calmer surroundings. A study using this unique nature soundtrack at Mayo Clinic with patients who had undergone open heart surgery showed that it helped them relax and manage their pain.

Other studies done at various research institutions resonate with these findings. One study found that indoor biophilic elements helped reduce blood pressure and improve short-term memory. Participants also reported a decrease in negative emotions and an increase in positive ones. Another study found that using houseplants and creating "virtual windows" in windowless locations to create an impression of the natural outdoors also had positive effects.

How to create your own biophilic environment
The trend in biophilic design in office spaces, medical institutions and even schools is increasing. It's also a pretty easy concept to implement in your personal spaces. Here are some suggestions for creating a biophilic oasis in your own bedroom or living room.

- Introduce or add houseplants to your home. Even artificial plants bring a sense of greenery.
- Consider growing herbs such as basil, chives and parsley. If you don't have adequate natural lighting, there are relatively inexpensive grow lights available that you can place over your plants.
- Add a small fountain or water feature in your home, or play sounds of a waterfall on a speaker.
- Immerse yourself in nature's scenery and sounds by displaying videos of natural environments on a digital screen, such as a TV or digital tablet.
- Complete the immersion by adding natural scents such as lavender or lemongrass. (Read more about aromatherapy on page 80.)
- If you're a pet owner, you have a built-in biophilic element. To get the benefits of fauna in your home, you don't necessarily need a dog or cat. Lower-maintenance pets such as fish or a gecko also give you opportunities to pause and observe life.

Wellness during illness

If you think holistic health is only for young and beautiful influencers on social media, think again. In real life, it doesn't matter whether you're 20 and running marathons or 50 and managing diabetes. Regardless of your current state of health, there's almost always one thing you can do to increase your well-being and quality of life. In fact, a holistic approach to your health may bring even more benefits when you're coping with an illness.

Everyone experiences illness at one point or another. And with age, illnesses often become chronic.

Today's healthcare system directs people to bring these issues to primary care professionals who are trained in treating disease — providing medications, procedures and therapy to reverse, stabilize or improve health conditions. This is often helpful.

But a holistic vision of healthcare takes a slightly different approach. Rather than focus solely on treating a person's disease, a holistic view aims to improve all aspects of that person's health. For example, suppose your hands ache from arthritis and you're unable to sleep. Your primary care team's first instinct might be to prescribe some medications to ease the pain.

But an integrative medicine approach considers a broader range of therapies to create a holistic treatment plan — and seeks to maximize overall quality of life. Alongside medication, you and your healthcare team might consider other therapies — such as gentle exercises, mind-body techniques or sauna use — to relieve symptoms of arthritis.

More and more people are looking for ways to manage illness and live better that don't involve taking so many medications, with all their attending side effects, or going through invasive medical procedures.

Instead, many of these people are looking for options that ease disease symptoms but also increase overall wellness. They want therapies that bring calm, improve sleep, boost mood and generally make them more resilient to life's stressors. They want to mend not only physical or mental problems but also themselves as a whole.

PUTTING YOUR INNATE HEALING POWERS TO WORK

Fusing the powers of mind, body and spirit can be a potent tool to mediate the symptoms of disease and find ways to enjoy life even when living with a chronic condition. Research finds that the human mind can be incredibly powerful in tuning the body to achieve greater resilience and better healing.

Many of the everyday things we take for granted — such as taking a deep breath, pausing to observe a detail or spending time in nature — can be powerful wellness boosters. Just a few years ago, getting a massage or relaxing in a hot tub was considered pampering or merely an enjoyable activity. But now scientists understand that these actions can have big effects on heart rate, metabolism, immune function, respiratory rate, muscle and joint health, and more. Many of these holistic therapies also produce positive effects on the brain, stimulating the release of the feel-good chemicals that act as stress reducers. Essentially, we all come with built-in self-healing talents; we just need to learn to use them.

Research finds that holistic practices are growing in popularity in many areas of medicine, including chronic disease management. Chronic illnesses take a substantial physical and mental toll, not just in terms of symptoms but also often in terms of treatment side effects. A holistic approach to disease management considers all aspects of a condition and how that sum total affects a person's life. The goal is to help lift that burden by improving the person's quality of life in addition to managing disease symptoms.

Cancer treatment leads the way

Cancer treatment is an example of a medical field in which the use of holistic therapies is rapidly increasing. Worldwide, rates of cancer continue to grow. Modern treatments improve survival, which means that more people are living with a history of cancer. In fact, estimates say

Wellness during illness **51**

WHAT HOLISTIC HEALTH LOOKS LIKE

Part of taking a holistic approach to health is recognizing that each person has their own unique health needs and goals. As a result, different therapies might help different people. Here are some scenarios illustrating how a holistic health approach may work, depending on life circumstances and individual preferences. Let these examples inspire you to consider therapies that might enhance your own health.

JULIA is a new mother working on her college degree online. She is healthy and energetic, and she wants to make sure she stays fit and socially engaged while taking care of her child and working on her degree. Between parenting and classes, she can't go out to exercise as often as she'd like to, and she wants to be more connected to people in her community. Julia is trying various exercises she can do at home, such as yoga, qigong and Pilates. When she is out with her baby, she takes long walks in parks. And she is discussing with her healthcare team whether she should take any vitamins or supplements now that she's had her baby. Julia is also an animal lover and has a dog. She is considering volunteering with her dog for the animal-assisted services at her local hospital.

SHOSHANA is 38 and is living with multiple sclerosis. Her medications are helping, but they also have side effects. She feels fatigued and exhausted much of the time. She wants to help her husband take care of their three young children. After discussing her options with her healthcare team, Shoshana is staying on her medications, but she's also going to try several nondrug approaches to reduce pain and fatigue. She is planning to sign up for yoga classes and try qigong. She read that cryotherapy, the therapeutic use of cold, might help reduce inflammation in people with multiple sclerosis. She is interested in trying it, so she's discussing it with her doctor. Cryotherapy is expensive, but she feels that if it works, it might be worth it.

MOHAMMAD is a busy 58-year-old executive at a fast-growing startup. He's recently been diagnosed with early-stage colon cancer and his treatment plan includes surgery and chemotherapy. He is divorced and his children live far away. Since he lives alone and plans to keep working as much as he can during treatment, Mohammad feels he must focus on maintaining his strength and energy levels. To bolster his physical strength and endurance, he started Pilates and tai chi. Mohammad also enjoys listening to music and plays the violin. He began regularly listening to classical music to reduce stress and practices deep breathing while listening. It's a good option for him, because he can do it during his workday in between meetings and phone calls. He is discussing with his healthcare team whether acupuncture and probiotics may help him with nausea and digestive issues as he goes through chemotherapy.

 BOB AND MARY have been married for 40 years and are retiring. Bob has heart disease and high blood pressure, and Mary has rheumatoid arthritis and fibromyalgia. At the community center they belong to, Bob and Mary have access to hot tubs and a sauna. These are good options for them because warm water often soothes aches and pains and may even reduce blood pressure. And a sauna session can elevate heart rate in a way similar to exercise. Bob and Mary also enjoy massage, but frequent massage sessions can get expensive. They plan to learn a few basic massage techniques so they can give massages to each other. They also plan to start taking regular walks at their local nature conservation area to fulfill the "park prescription" they received from their family doctor. They're reading about the benefits of forest bathing and are planning to install an herb and vegetable garden in their backyard.

that by 2040, about 26 million people will be either living with cancer or living as a cancer survivor. Many cancer survivors cope with physical and mental challenges on a daily basis, and that's where holistic therapies can help.

A survey of more than 1,000 patients and 150 cancer specialists found that over 60% of cancer patients strongly believe in holistic therapies, and a similar percentage used at least one such practice. More than 70% want their healthcare systems to offer such therapies, and more than half say that they would've chosen a healthcare system that offers holistic therapies if they could go back in time.

Medical professionals are on board too. Among cancer specialists, over half believe that holistic therapies are effective at managing treatment side effects and a third believe that these therapies improve overall survival. Nearly all cancer care institutions now offer at least one type of holistic therapy as part of a comprehensive treatment plan.

WHY TAKE A HOLISTIC APPROACH?

There are growing reasons why more and more people are exploring holistic living. They want to not only manage chronic illnesses successfully but also to live longer, happier lives.

Readily available research
People today are much better at educating themselves about their illnesses and overall wellness. Two decades ago, consumers had little access to research or reliable medical information. Today, information about clinical trials and pharmaceutical developments is widely available to the public. Online search engines allow anyone with internet access to research diseases and conditions, medication side effects, surgical options and nondrug alternatives. People are also taking a more active role in their own healthcare, and many would like to have options that are less invasive or have fewer side effects.

Chronic stress management
Holistic medicine offers several effective, evidence-based approaches to dealing with stress and illness that can complement a medical treatment plan. Taking a prescribed medication may help bring your blood pressure level into a healthy range, but adding meditation to your daily wellness routine may stop your blood pressure from spiking to begin

---

54   Mayo Clinic Guide to Holistic Health

The Society for Integrative Oncology recommends the following therapies as part of cancer treatment:

- Mindfulness
- Yoga
- Relaxation techniques
- Music therapy
- Reflexology
- Aromatherapy
- Acupuncture
- Tai chi
- Qigong

You can read more about these kinds of interventions in the "Therapies A–Z" section.

with — and prevent you from needing to take a second medication. Many people are learning to manage the stress in their lives successfully by using mind-body methods such as yoga, meditation, massage and guided imagery.

Baby boomer interest
Baby boomers today are often dealing with multiple medical issues, such as weight management, joint pain, high blood pressure and elevated cholesterol. With the growing awareness that pills aren't always the answer, baby boomers are actively exploring other ways to age well. Not everyone wants to start with medication; many prefer to tackle their issues noninvasively, at least at first — by changing their diets, exercising and managing stress, for example.

Cost efficiency and ease
Many holistic therapies can be not only medically effective but also cost effective. Participating in a yoga class or meditating at home can be significantly cheaper than taking a medication that insurance may or may not cover. And you remain in control of your options at all times — you don't need a prescription to switch from tai chi to Pilates or to take regular walks in the park.

BALANCING MEDICINE AND WELLNESS

There's no doubt that medical treatments save millions of lives every year. If it wasn't for antibiotics, for example, hundreds of thousands of adults and children would still be dying from common infections, as they were before such drugs were invented. People with diabetes would have much lower life expectancy without insulin. More and more people are able to survive cancer thanks to surgery, chemotherapy and radiation therapy. Medicines also enable individuals with chronic conditions to live longer, more active lives.

The problem with too much medicine

But drugs and procedures can only go so far in promoting health. And sometimes they can even take away from health. Many Americans, particularly older adults who are often dealing with several health issues at once, are taking a multitude of pills. Between 1988 and 2010 the average number of prescription medications taken by those over 65 doubled and the proportion of those taking more than five medications tripled.

Called polypharmacy, the practice of taking multiple drugs may be problematic for several reasons. All drugs carry the potential for side effects, and some drugs can cause bad side effects. Some drugs interact with each other, reducing their effectiveness or maybe even causing harm. And when you have so many pills to keep track of, it can be easy to mix up regimens or forget to take some.

Conventional medicine has often relied on the belief that medications are the best and easiest approach for treating many conditions, from metabolic disorders to mental health to chronic pain. What can be easier than taking a pill? But that approach is not without difficulties. Too often, people's health challenges are addressed as problems to be fixed quickly and cheaply rather than as multilayered needs, including those of an emotional and spiritual nature. As a result, people may end up feeling overwhelmed by the myriad tests and drugs offered to them as healthcare.

No quick fixes

Although the quick-fix approach can be efficient in simple cases, today scientists no longer think it works across the board.

Opioids are a poignant example of medicine that was meant to help people in pain but ended up also causing untold harm. Opioid overuse led to addictions, overdoses and deaths. Of the more than 70,000 drug overdose deaths in the United States in 2017, approximately two-thirds involved an opioid. Drug overdose deaths rose from 2019 to 2021, with more than 106,000 deaths reported in 2021. Opioid misuse in adults over 65 in particular has risen sharply. One study reported a 220% increase in opioid misuse in this population.

56   Mayo Clinic Guide to Holistic Health

> # As distressing as life-changing events are, they can come with a sliver of a silver lining, even if it's not apparent at first.

Scientists and physicians also are finding that medications can artificially restructurethe body's metabolism in ways that have unknown or unintended consequences. Drugs that alter aspects of the body's metabolism may affect how other organs work. It also may force the body into trying to compensate for the changes in other ways — and throw something else out of balance. Lastly, taking certain drugs for years may have long-term consequences that don't become apparent until decades later.

One of the hard-earned lessons from the opioid epidemic is that pills aren't always the solution they were meant to be. In the United States and across the world, scientists are reframing their approach to treating pain and disease, increasingly embracing a more holistic, whole-person approach to health.

LIVING WELL DESPITE DISCOMFORT OR PAIN

Mayo Clinic cardiologist Stephen Kopecky, M.D., knows how challenging it can be to deal with a life-threatening illness. Dr. Kopecky was first diagnosed with cancer during his rotations as a medical student. He was cured after a surgery and six weeks of radiation. As a young man in pursuit of a medical career, he put the episode behind him.

Less than two decades later, cancer returned in a more aggressive form, now spreading through his body. Dr. Kopecky realized that having cancer twice before he even turned 40 greatly increased his odds of developing other health problems in the future. Following successful treatment of the second cancer, he made the decision to have the best health possible for as long as possible. "In other words, I wanted to live younger longer," he later wrote in his book by the same title, *Live Younger Longer*. So he learned everything he could do to prevent future cancer and major diseases from taking hold.

As distressing as life-changing events are, they can come with a sliver of a silver lining, even if it's not apparent at first. Realizing exactly how much your health matters to you makes you want to renew your commitment to health and do everything possible to avoid diseases in the future. "A healthy person has a thousand wishes, a sick person only

QUESTIONS TO ASK YOUR HEALTHCARE TEAM ABOUT A NEW MEDICINE

If you're being prescribed a new medicine, it's OK to ask questions so that you know why you're taking it and understand the medicine's risks and benefits. Ask your healthcare team, including your pharmacist:

- What is the name of the medicine and why am I taking it?
- What medical condition does this medicine treat?
- How do I know if the medicine is working?
- What type of side effects might I expect, if any? What should I do if I experience serious side effects?
- Will this drug cause problems if I am taking other prescriptions, over-the-counter medicines or supplements?
- What should I do if I want to stop taking this medicine? Is it safe to stop abruptly?
- Are there nonpharmaceutical alternatives or lifestyle interventions that might help my condition? What about complementary therapies?
- Is it safe for me to drive while taking this medication?
- Should I take the medicine with food or not? Is there anything I should not eat or drink when taking this medicine?
- What does "take as needed" mean?
- If I forget to take my medicine, what should I do?
- How will this medicine affect all the other drugs I am taking?

When you live with a chronic condition, it's important to trust your healthcare team. But it's also important to understand all aspects of your treatment plan and ask questions about anything you don't understand.

By the same token, it's important for you to be transparent with your healthcare team about any holistic therapies you're using or contemplating, so that they can take these therapies into account when considering your overall treatment plan.

For example, if your pain medication's side effects are bothering you, you and your primary care provider might decide to do a trial of massage therapy. If massage proves helpful, you might be able to decrease or eliminate your pain medication.

58   Mayo Clinic Guide to Holistic Health

one," says the traditional proverb. It is often during those darkest moments of our health journeys that we make life-altering decisions to take better care of ourselves.

Dr. Kopecky cites a curious paradigm. William Mosley, who was the chief of medicine at John Hopkins University about a century ago, famously said that the secret to a long life is getting a chronic disease — and taking good care of it. That counterintuitive statement comes with hidden wisdom. Having a medical problem often forces you to confront your health and make necessary changes, such as ditching bad habits and developing healthy ones.

Embrace *your* health

In a roundabout way, disease can steer you toward a more holistic lifestyle. That more holistic way of living can bring more benefits than overcoming the disease itself or learning to live with it. It can push you to change how you live, eat, sleep, exercise and deal with stress. And it can reduce the chances of developing future diseases. You can use your illness to take better care of yourself, so you not only manage your condition but also enjoy your life in total.

Take charge
If you're living with a long-term or life-threatening illness, knowing about your disease can help you manage it. The more you learn, the more in control you will begin to feel — rather than feeling like your disease is controlling you.

- **Research your condition** Ask your healthcare team for trustworthy websites to visit, as not all online information is reliable.
- **Reach out to others with similar conditions** Join a support group or national organization or find a social network.
- **Maintain a positive attitude** Studies find that optimistic people not only deal better with stress and setbacks but even live longer.

Use your illness as a catalyst for personal growth
It's often tempting to feel resentful about your disease and focus on what you can't do. But try to look for opportunities to widen your outlook and promote your health.
- Accept the limitations of your illness.
- Make a list of your current strengths, what you're good at.
- Look for ways to apply your strengths and develop them.
- Give back to others, using your talents.

Think outside the box
Use this book to help you explore a more holistic approach to your health.

Find out more about different complementary therapies in the "Therapies A–Z" section. For example:

- To reduce stress and improve mood, try meditation, mindfulness, music therapy or aromatherapy.
- To reduce pain and fatigue, try massage, acupuncture or sauna.
- To boost strength, energy and endurance, try yoga, tai chi or qigong.
- Speak to your healthcare team about other forms of holistic therapies that might help with your condition.

LOOKING AHEAD

In the 20th century, medicine focused on finding therapies that worked effectively for as many people as possible. Think antibiotics, fever reducers and vaccines. In the 21st century, the focus is increasingly on the individual. As science realizes that every person has a unique microbiome, set of genes and life experiences that dictate how they may respond to treatments, it is becoming clear that health is best addressed at the individual level. That field is now known as personalized medicine.

Data and tools to help physicians provide personalized care with better precision are already in the works. For example, the Human Genome Project, completed in 2003, delivered a detailed map of our genetic makeup. Similarly, the Human Microbiome Project sequenced the human microbiome, informing us of what microorganisms live in and on us and how they affect our health.

Yet while we know what some of our genes do, we still don't have a clear picture of how they all function. And science has yet to figure out what an optimal microbiome looks like, and whether that varies by individual. Newly developed artificial intelligence tools can plow through vast quantities of information to help scientists make sense of all these tremendous complexities.

The future is personalized

The hope is that there will come a time when medical professionals look at a person's genome, microbiome and other information to identify that person's unique health profile. This might include genetic susceptibilities to various diseases as well as health-related strengths such as protective genes or beneficial metabolic factors.

If medicine becomes more adept at fusing ancient medical knowledge and experience with modern high-tech science, a better and more holistic approach to health may emerge. For example, physicians might be able to deduce from a person's data what probiotics the person needs. Or whether, compared with the experience of thousands of

The more you learn, the more in control you will begin to feel.

others with similar profiles, the person could benefit from a specific, directed therapy.

It will take time to get there. But the good news is that you don't have to wait for this to happen to start your own personalized health journey. You can use this book to learn how to approach your health in a holistic way that works for you — one that builds on whole-health fundamentals and uses therapies that best fit your lifestyle and goals to further enhance your physical, emotional and spiritual wellness.

PART 2

Therapies
A–Z

Acupuncture

Acupuncture involves the insertion of very thin needles through your skin at strategic points on your body to stimulate health. Historical mention of acupuncture dates to 2600 B.C.E. in China, when fine-sharpened stone or bamboo needles were used to treat various illnesses. Over time, the practice has spread around the world. The word *acupuncture* is derived from the Latin words *acus* (needle) and *punctura* (penetration).

In the United States, the use of acupuncture can be traced back to the 18th century, when it was mentioned in a medical text. However, it didn't enter the mainstream until 1971, when *New York Times* journalist James Reston visited China and wrote about how acupuncture helped relieve his postoperative pain. His experience piqued Western interest.

Over the past few decades, research into acupuncture as a medical treatment has grown exponentially. More than 13,000 studies have been conducted in 60 countries, examining acupuncture as a therapy for pain, pregnancy, stroke, mood disorders, sleep disorders, inflammation and many other conditions.

Today, acupuncture is one of the most commonly available therapies worldwide. According to the World Health Organization, it is used in 103 of 129 countries that reported data. An estimated 3 million American adults receive acupuncture each year.

In some cases, the therapy seems to have long-lasting positive effects. An analysis of data from 20 studies and several thousand patients dealing with painful conditions — such as headaches, osteoarthritis and back and neck pain — showed that the beneficial effects of acupuncture lasted even after the sessions were stopped, in many cases up to a year.

WHY IT'S DONE

Acupuncture is used mainly to relieve discomfort associated with a variety of conditions, including:

- Neck pain.
- Lower back pain.
- Osteoarthritis.
- Headaches, including tension headaches and migraines.
- Chemotherapy-induced and postoperative nausea and vomiting.
- Fibromyalgia.
- Labor pain.
- Menstrual cramps.

DIFFERENT VANTAGE POINTS

The Western view of how acupuncture works differs somewhat from traditional Chinese beliefs. Western practitioners view acupoints, where needles are placed, as places to stimulate nerves, muscles and connective tissue. Some believe that this sensory stimulation increases blood flow and boosts your body's natural painkillers — endogenous opioid peptides called endorphins. Both Western and traditional Chinese views agree that acupuncture can be an efficient way to relieve pain for some people. It also seems to have an overall positive effect on health and well-being.

- Respiratory disorders, such as allergic rhinitis.
- Tennis elbow.
- Dental pain.

HOW IT WORKS

According to traditional Chinese medicine theory, the human body contains energy channels or pathways called meridians, which wind through the body like rivers, nourishing its organs and tissues. Through these channels, it is believed, flows the vital energy or life force called qi (CHEE). Qi is thought to bring balance to various aspects of your health, including your spiritual, emotional, mental and physical health.

A blockage in your meridians acts like a dam that backs up water, preventing qi from reaching and nourishing the organs. Stimulating specific spots on the meridians called acupoints removes the blockage and restores the flow of qi. According to traditional Chinese medicine, the human body contains 14 energy meridians with 400 acupoints distributed across them. Acupuncture needles are used to stimulate these acupoints.

A common misconception about acupuncture is that it's a stand-alone treatment. Acupuncture is usually one of several components that make up a larger treatment program. To begin treatment, most traditional Chinese medicine practitioners take a detailed history of the person being treated and will check the person's tongue and pulse. (A Western practitioner may do so as well, but the traditional Chinese medicine approach is more detailed.)

Traditional Chinese medicine practitioners check the tongue because it's considered an important diagnostic tool. Certain areas of the tongue correlate with particular areas of the body. Your practitioner also may carefully examine the shape, coating and color of your tongue.

Another diagnostic tool, important in both Western and Chinese medicine, is your pulse. Traditional Chinese medicine has an elaborate system of diagnosis based on characteristics of the pulse. Your acupuncture practitioner may examine its strength, rhythm and quality.

"We use observations of the tongue and pulse as components of our diagnosis, along with the information that the person shares with us and

EXPERT INSIGHT
AN OPTION FOR CANCER CARE

Molly J. Mallory, L.Ac., an acupuncturist at Mayo Clinic, is accustomed to treating cancer patients struggling with side effects of their cancer or cancer treatment. One case she remembers vividly: a young woman in her early 40s going through treatment for breast cancer. A tailor by profession, she was suffering from pain in her hands so severe that she could no longer work. She also struggled with fatigue and nausea and her symptoms made it difficult to participate in family activities.

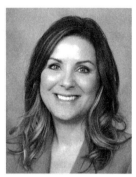

Molly J. Mallory, L.Ac.
Integrative Medicine and Health

After a series of acupuncture treatments, the pain relented and she was able to return to work. "Not only did it give her joy but it gave her an income again," Mallory says. "She was so happy. I've seen similar results with many oncology patients. They are finding relief from symptoms such as nausea, fatigue, digestive upset, insomnia and anxiety — which increases their quality of life."

"I think that patients are driving the increase in doctors' referrals for acupuncture," Mallory says. As a practitioner, Mallory has seen acupuncture work on many different conditions. It's particularly effective at alleviating pain, which makes it a potential alternative to opioids for people with chronic pain. Increasingly, people are interested in pain treatments that have fewer side effects, or even positive side effects, and that contribute to a more holistic approach.

the person's Western medical diagnosis, to formulate the Chinese medical diagnosis," says Molly J. Mallory, L.Ac., an acupuncturist at Mayo Clinic. "That aids us in determining the treatment plan and acupoint selection, as well as lifestyle modification suggestions."

After gathering all the necessary information, the acupuncturist develops a holistic plan to restore the body's balance. That plan will likely include acupuncture, but it also may include recommendations about diet, lifestyle, herbs, massage or exercises such as tai chi or qigong.

PREPARING FOR ACUPUNCTURE

On the day of your acupuncture treatment, there are some things you can do to prepare yourself. This advice comes from the American Academy of Medical Acupuncture, the professional society of physicians in North America who have incorporated acupuncture into their traditional medical practice.

- Don't eat an unusually large meal right before or after your treatment.
- Don't exercise vigorously, engage in sexual activity or consume alcoholic beverages within six hours before or after treatment. Alcohol and vigorous activities may counteract the effects of acupuncture.
- Try to avoid caffeine for 2 to 4 hours before the treatment, as it can counteract the treatment effects.
- Plan your activities so that after your treatment you can get some rest — or at least not have to be working at top performance. This is especially important for the first few visits.
- Continue to take any prescription medicines as directed by your healthcare team.
- Remember to keep good notes of your response to each treatment session so that follow-up sessions can be refined based on your feedback.

WORKING WITH A PRACTITIONER

If you're considering acupuncture therapy, it's important to find a qualified practitioner. Most states license acupuncturists, but the requirements for licensing vary from state to state. Take the same steps you might take to choose any other medical professional:

- Ask people you trust for recommendations.
- Check the practitioner's training and credentials. Most states require that acupuncturists who aren't physicians pass an exam conducted by the National Certification Commission for Acupuncture and Oriental Medicine.
- Interview the practitioner. Ask what's involved in the treatment, how likely it is to help your condition and how much it will cost.

- Find out whether your insurance covers the treatment. Some health insurance policies cover acupuncture, but others don't. Coverage is often limited based on the condition being treated. For example, Medicare currently covers acupuncture only for the treatment of chronic low back pain. Medicaid coverage of acupuncture varies from state to state.

WHAT TO EXPECT DURING ACUPUNCTURE

Each person who performs acupuncture has a unique style and may blend aspects of Eastern and Western approaches to medicine. To help determine the type of acupuncture treatment that may help you the most, your practitioner may ask you about your symptoms, behaviors and lifestyle.

Your acupuncture practitioner will tell you the general site of the planned treatment and whether you need to remove any clothing. A gown, towel or sheet will generally be provided. You lie on a padded table for the treatment.

Many people wonder where the needles will be placed. Acupuncture points are located all over the body. Sometimes the appropriate points are far removed from the area of your pain. It's OK to ask your practitioner where the needles will be placed in your specific case. Treatments can last from 30 minutes to an hour, with the needles being retained for 15 to 20 minutes, or sometimes up to half an hour.

Most people who receive acupuncture feel only minimal sensation as the needles are inserted; some feel no sensation at all. "Some people describe their sensation as tingling or heaviness," Mallory shares. "That's because acupuncture uses different, much thinner needles than the traditional hypodermic ones used to inject medicine. They are about as thin as a human hair. They sort of glide into the tissue rather than breaking or causing any damage to the tissue."

Your practitioner may gently move or twirl the needles after placement or apply heat or mild electrical pulses to the needles. A low-intensity electric current may be applied to some needles to add stimulation. Another technique your practitioner may use is moxibustion, in which an herb is burned near the acupuncture point or on the needle itself.

At Mayo Clinic, a typical acupuncture visit takes 45 to 60 minutes, during which the patient rests with the needles for 20 to 30 minutes. The placement and number of needles depend on the health condition being treated and the patient's general state of health. An average number of needles can range from 10 to 20. "The treatments are really individualized," Mallory says. "We have music playing, we dim the lights and we have relaxing nature scenery on a television screen. We also have infrared heat lamps to keep patients warm and comfortable or to help with musculoskeletal conditions."

After an acupuncture treatment, most people feel intense relaxation, due to the endorphins released. That is particularly pronounced with the first session or two.

Because acupuncture is individually tailored to each patient, the frequency and duration of therapies differ. In general, most conditions can be treated with 6 to 12 sessions of acupuncture.

Because acupuncture practitioners work very closely with their patients while placing needles, acupuncture sessions can offer additional diagnostic capabilities. In several cases, during therapy sessions Mayo Clinic acupuncturists and massage therapists found suspicious formations or masses on their patients' bodies and referred them to imaging procedures. The tests found cancer, which otherwise could have remained undetected for longer.

> ### ACUPUNCTURE AT MAYO CLINIC
>
> Acupuncture has been used at Mayo Clinic since the mid-1990s. Mayo Clinic's licensed acupuncture specialists perform more than 1,400 acupuncture treatments each year.

RESEARCH ON ACUPUNCTURE

Researchers continue to study acupuncture to find out how it works from a scientific perspective and to see how effective it might be to treat certain conditions.

Clinical trials of acupuncture's effectiveness can be challenging because a well-designed trial needs a placebo for comparison. Research studies often use a sugar pill or saline injection for a placebo, but in acupuncture, it's more difficult to have a true placebo to test against. Even with this challenge, evidence indicates that acupuncture is effective for certain conditions and certain people.

Pain

Treatment for pain is the best-studied aspect of acupuncture. The processing of pain signals involves many parts of the brain. In addition, how much pain you feel partly depends on the context. Our body's natural painkillers — known as endogenous opioids — may play a key role in how acupuncture helps treat pain.

Researchers at the University of Michigan found that acupuncture increases the number of opioid receptors in the brain. These structures play a key role in pain relief. Evidence supports the idea that opioid peptides are released during acupuncture, and the pain-relieving effects of acupuncture are at least partially explained by the actions of these substances.

Other research has shown that acupuncture can help treat different types of pain: chronic neck pain, chronic and acute low back pain, knee pain, dental pain, osteoarthritis, labor pain, sciatica, menstrual cramps and headaches, including migraine headaches. Scientists also found that acupuncture can produce anti-inflammatory effects by balancing out immune system functions.

Fibromyalgia

Investigators at Mayo Clinic focused on acupuncture and fibromyalgia, a disorder that involves widespread musculoskeletal pain accompanied by fatigue, sleep, memory and mood issues. In the study, the researchers gave one group of people true acupuncture while the other received a brief poke by a toothpick done with a visual barrier so they couldn't see whether the needles were placed or not.

One month later, the group that received the true acupuncture showed a reduction in their Fibromyalgia Impact Questionnaire (FIQ) scores, a standard method of measuring fibromyalgia symptoms. These participants also felt less anxiety and pain. Six months later, the group that received true acupuncture still showed a meaningful reduction in pain, anxiety and FIQ scores.

Back pain

Back pain is a common reason for visits to licensed acupuncturists because many people who are dissatisfied with more mainstream treatments seek alternatives. Several recent studies have suggested that both real acupuncture and "sham" acupuncture (the shallow needling of points) are equally effective for treating chronic low back pain, and that both can be part of medical care.

Cancer and chemotherapy side effects

Acupuncture can reduce nausea and vomiting in people who are receiving chemotherapy, which helps them keep food down — and therefore improves their nutrition intake.

Acupuncture also may help ease pain caused by cancer and chemotherapy. Whether caused by tumors or treatments such as surgery, chemotherapy and radiation, pain is one of the most common and debilitating symptoms that affect people with cancer. Pain can be acute or chronic, and often it is resistant to conventional interventions. After analyzing 227 relevant studies conducted and published between 1990 and 2021, Mayo Clinic researchers concluded that acupuncture can be effective at alleviating joint, musculoskeletal and general cancer pain.

"Many of my oncology patients are experiencing nausea, anxiety, digestive issues and insomnia," Mallory says. "Some also have tingling,

> The Evidence Based Acupuncture Project found acupuncture to be an effective treatment for a range of medical problems including digestive disorders, respiratory disorders, neurological and muscular disorders, and urinary and menstrual problems.

numbness and pain in their hands and feet. There aren't a lot of good Western medicine treatments for some of those things. So sometimes when patients come in for acupuncture, they're so incredibly relieved. Some of them say, 'This is the first time I didn't get really sick and nauseous after chemo.' Or 'This is the first time I wasn't in bed for three days after chemotherapy.' Or 'This is the first time I slept through the night.'"

Heart health

A recent Mayo Clinic study used acupuncture to reduce the incidents of irregular heartbeat, called arrhythmia, in people recovering from cardiac surgery. Researchers administered acupuncture to 138 people and found that it not only reduced arrhythmia but also decreased blood pressure and lowered heart rate.

Fertility and pregnancy

Acupuncture may be effective for increasing fertility. It also may help maintain a healthy pregnancy and minimize nausea and fatigue. Toward the end of pregnancy, it can reduce back pain. It also can help induce and stimulate labor, as an alternative to medications or a C-section. "Acupuncture practitioners are trained on proper technique and which acupuncture points to use or avoid during pregnancy," Mallory says.

Spinal stenosis

Researchers have evaluated acupuncture in people with spinal stenosis — a condition in which degenerative changes in the bones and joints cause pinching on the spinal cord or spinal nerves, resulting in pain. Often age-related, it can worsen with time and result in surgery for some people. A recent study suggests that acupuncture can alleviate spinal stenosis pain on par with surgical interventions, offering a possible noninvasive alternative.

Other health conditions
There is evidence that acupuncture may help relieve seasonal allergy symptoms, and that it can help address incontinence in women. It also may help relieve symptoms and improve the quality of life in people with asthma, but it has not been shown to improve lung function. Acupuncture may provide relief from osteoarthritis and rheumatoid arthritis pain, and even ease depression caused by post-traumatic stress disorder.

RISKS AND SAFETY CONCERNS
The risks of acupuncture are low if you're working with a competent, certified acupuncture practitioner. A survey of 760,000 treatment sessions involving over 97,000 people in Germany found that only about 3% of them complained of pain and bruises caused by needles. A Japanese survey of over 65,000 acupuncture treatments reported no major adverse events. Two surveys performed in the United Kingdom totaling 66,000 treatments similarly didn't report any major problems. Single-use, disposable needles are now the practice standard, so the risk of infection is minimal.

There are times when acupuncture may not be advisable. Talk to your healthcare team if you:
- **Have a bleeding disorder** You may experience increased risk of bleeding or bruising from the needles if you have a bleeding disorder or if you're taking blood thinners.
- **Have a pacemaker** When acupuncture involves applying mild electrical pulses to the needles, this can interfere with a pacemaker's operation.
- **Are pregnant** Some acupoints on your body may stimulate labor. They should be avoided if you are pregnant.

OUR TAKE
Acupuncture can be effective when used alone or when added to other medical treatments. The Evidence Based Acupuncture Project, which covered nearly 1,000 systematic reviews of the practice, found acupuncture to be an effective treatment for a range of medical problems including digestive disorders, such as constipation; respiratory disorders, such as allergic rhinitis; neurological and muscular disorders, such as headache, stroke and neck pain; low back pain and sciatica; and urinary and menstrual problems. Generally, when administered by a qualified practitioner, acupuncture is considered safe.

Animal-assisted services

A 21-year-old Mayo Clinic patient with autism could not bring himself to tolerate chemotherapy for his nasopharynx cancer. The hospital settings, the needles and the feeling sick afterward overwhelmed his senses. Finally, his anxiety and his fear of the procedure escalated to the point that he had to be restrained, and it took four nurses to hold him.

One day, the nurses noticed how his behavior changed when he spotted a yellow Labrador named Lily in the clinic. Lily is a therapy dog who is part of Mayo Clinic's Caring Canine Program, and she is trained to provide comfort and support for patients. At home the young man had a yellow Labrador whom he loved very much, and Lily looked just like his dog. The nurses wondered whether Lily could help him get through the difficult procedure.

When the young man came for his next appointment, Lily and her volunteer handler came into the room. As soon as he saw the dog, his behavior changed. The nurses told him that Lily was there to help him get through the procedure, but she could stay only if he could keep them both safe. "Can you promise not to kick your legs? If you need to kick them, we'll have to leave," Lily's handler explained. The young man mustered his courage and responded, "I can do this."

As he received his chemotherapy, the young man petted Lily and talked about his dogs at home. His anxiety subsided and he was much calmer. He didn't need to be restrained at all. The nurses adjusted his schedule so that Lily could always accompany him for his chemotherapy appointments. "It was amazing," says Whitney Romine, animal-assisted services coordinator at Mayo Clinic, what a dog's presence could do for the patient. "He felt empowered enough to get himself through that."

TAPPING INTO AN ANCIENT BOND

The young man's story is a great example of animal-assisted services, also called animal-assisted treatment, animal-assisted support or previously, pet therapy. All these terms have a similar definition: programs that utilize specially trained animals to provide comfort and positive distraction for people in need. At Mayo Clinic, this includes patients and their families, as well as staff.

Animal-assisted services are a growing part of holistic care, particularly in hospital settings. They tap into the concept of human-animal bonds that date back to antiquity and have been documented throughout history. In ancient times, animals were essential partners in human survival, health and healing. Many spiritual traditions worldwide have honored relationships between people and animals.

Today, animals are assisting with patient care in various ways. Like Lily, animals can provide comfort and emotional support. They can nudge people to participate in rehabilitative activities, such as throwing a ball, walking up and down stairs, or bending down to do some petting. "I've seen physical therapists position the dog a certain way so the person has to bend and reach to pet the dog," says Romine. Such movement helps to restore mobility and flexibility.

Animal-assisted services also can help outside the hospital, such as by soothing and distracting older adults in long-term care facilities or military veterans dealing with post-traumatic stress disorder.

WHAT THE RESEARCH SHOWS

Stress contributes to many medical and mental health conditions. Animal-assisted services help reduce stress and promote relaxation. Animals also bring a sense of companionship, which reduces feelings of loneliness and social isolation. Some forms of animal-assisted support may even help reduce blood pressure. The physiologic effects of petting an animal include increases in serotonin, dopamine, prolactin and oxytocin — the "happiness hormones."

Modern research finds that animals can provide healing on many different levels. Here are some of the benefits animal companionship can provide:

- **Decreased stress and anxiety** Interacting with an animal can reduce stress, anxiety and depression; ease loneliness; and encourage exercise and playfulness. In a Mayo Clinic study of over 300 people who were receiving chemotherapy to treat advanced cancer, about half of the patients had pets. They felt less stressed and most of them said that their pets helped them cope.
- **Improved heart health** Animal companionship has been shown to reduce heart rate, blood pressure and triglyceride and cholesterol levels. A 2013 statement from the American Heart Association cited 81 different studies showing that having a pet helps in managing high blood pressure, high cholesterol and obesity.
- **Motivation to move** Having a pet can encourage the owner to exercise. On average, people who live with a dog walk one hour more per week compared to those who live without one.
- **Better quality of life** Pets enhance the quality of life, especially for older adults. They also boost the overall sense of wellness. In older adults, both loneliness and isolation were decreased for those who spent time with an animal. Elderly adults in nursing homes had better nutritional health when they ate their meals near an aquarium rather than alone.

- **Improved chronic illness coping skills** Pets have been shown to help people cope with chronic conditions and illnesses including heart disease, dementia and cancer, as well as developmental disabilities and mental health disorders, including depression, anxiety, attention-deficit/ hyperactivity disorder and schizophrenia. Interacting with an animal can help people with neurological diseases, both physically and mentally.

INTERESTED IN VOLUNTEERING WITH YOUR DOG?

Therapy dogs can provide joy and comfort in a healthcare setting to anyone who could use a smile, a little motivation or a lift in their spirits. If you're interested in teaming up with your dog to provide animal-assisted services, Romine offers the following tips.

Study your dog What body language does your dog use to communicate when they are stressed, neutral, calm or happy? How do you know when your dog doesn't feel well? Does your dog light up and curiously investigate new environments and people? Does your dog check in with you frequently and respond to your cues quickly? Make notes and create your own dog profile.

Think about where you would like to visit If you have a facility in mind where you would like to visit with your dog, give the staff a call. Ask if the facility has any special requirements, including registration through a specific therapy dog organization.

Practice with your dog The best therapy dog teams are the ones that have a strong bond created through a history of working together. Practicing helps strengthen that bond. You can practice by visiting close family or friends at home, and then friendly strangers in pet-friendly establishments. If you are planning on volunteering in a clinic, introduce your dog to items found in a hospital. Familiarize your dog with a wheelchair. Train your dog to interact with a person lying in bed. "Does your dog automatically jump on the bed without a cue from you? That can be a problem if they do that in a hospital and they accidentally jump on somebody who has a sore spot," Romine points out — but training can help. Therapy dog teams are often trained to be responsive to each other, and they can remain calm and comfortable in a variety of settings with a variety of people.

Take a class Take an all-positive, rewards-based class with your dog. Talk to the trainer to get another opinion of your dog's disposition, behavior and obedience level to see if your dog is a good fit for therapy work. Although it is not required, some owners find the American Kennel Club

EXPERT INSIGHT
ANIMAL-ASSISTED SERVICES AT MAYO CLINIC

You might say that Mayo Clinic has gone to the dogs — but that's not a bad thing.

That's because on Mayo Clinic's Minnesota, Arizona and Florida campuses, as many as 100 dogs are providing comfort to those in need as part of animal-assisted support services.

At Mayo Clinic, staff appreciate the value of the human-animal bond. Physicians may add a companion animal's name to a patient's file. After talking about medical issues the patient is facing, staff will shift the conversation to the elements of their life that bring them joy and purpose. They find that taking time to talk to patients about their furry family members and to arrange for a bedside visit at the end of life means more to patients and their families than can ever be put into words.

Currently, there are two programs at Mayo: Caring Canines and facility dogs.

Caring Canines

The Caring Canines program relies on a group of volunteers who have been registered with their dogs through a hospital-approved organization that educates, evaluates and registers therapy animal teams. Mayo Clinic has offered the Caring Canines program since the early 2000s in Rochester, and since 2011 in Arizona and Florida.

Where might you find therapy dogs working at Mayo Clinic?

There are very few places they *can't* go. Outpatient waiting rooms, hospitals, psychology and psychiatry areas, and physical therapy clinics are just some of the many places you might see a Caring Canines therapy dog.

They're also featured as part of structured group visits, and they go door-to-door to see patients. But that's not all — therapy dogs make the rounds at staff wellness events and even visit students to provide stress relief during midterms and finals.

"We go around and bring comfort and joy to patients and take their minds off of being stuck in the hospital," Romine says. "Almost every day, our volunteer teams will share a story about someone who connected with a Caring Canine and say, 'This is the best part of my day,' and it literally brings tears to their eyes," Romine says of her experiences supporting volunteer handlers in the Caring Canines program.

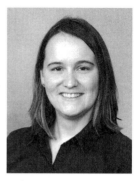

Whitney M. Romine
Animal-Assisted Services

Facility dogs
Facility dogs provide similar services for patients, but they go through a more robust training than a typical volunteer's dog. Bred and nurtured by a hospital-approved facility dog organization, facility dogs complete an extensive two-year program in which they learn skilled tasks to complement the work of a licensed clinician or professional. At the end of the program, facility dogs and their handlers are certified by an evaluator from a facility dog organization before they start helping humans.

Mayo Clinic piloted working with facility dogs in clinical care in 2019. They've since added additional facility dogs to their roster. Unlike the Caring Canine dogs, facility dogs are assigned to live with a Mayo Clinic employee. While therapy dogs come for short visits, facility dogs are "full-timers." "The facility dogs will work anywhere from 6 to 8 hours a day, whereas the therapy dogs will only work two as a maximum," says Romine. "They're kind of like an advanced-level therapy dog."

And while Caring Canines frequent many locations within the clinic, facility dogs are assigned to a specific unit within the hospital. They work in their assigned unit with the employee they are partnered with. For example, one of the Mayo Clinic's facility dogs only visits children at the General Pediatrics unit she is assigned to. And at the end of the day, these facility dogs go home with their assigned member of the Mayo Clinic staff.

Canine Good Citizen test to be a helpful way to measure their dog's baseline skills and see how their dog will respond in a more formal setting.

Join a reputable organization A reputable organization typically tests and registers therapy dog teams. It places the welfare of therapy animals as their highest priority, empowers handlers to advocate for their animal partners and provides liability insurance support to protect teams during their visits. Do your homework and choose the organization that fits you best.

Two well-known national therapy dog registries are:
- Alliance of Therapy Dogs: *www.therapydogs.com*
- Pet Partners: *www.petpartners.org*

ALL ABOUT THE DOGS
Therapy dogs, facility dogs, service dogs, emotional support dogs: What's the difference?

A **therapy dog** is a dog that goes with their handler to volunteer at schools, hospitals and nursing homes. From playing with small children to cuddling with a senior in assisted living, therapy dogs and their handlers work together as a team to improve the lives of other people.

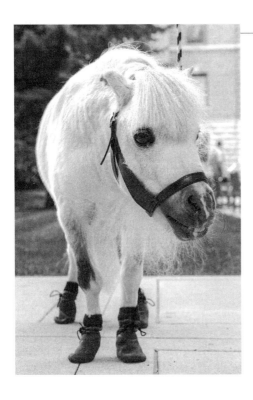

A MINI HORSE CALLED MUNCHKIN

Dogs aren't the only animals who provide therapy. Most recently, a horse with dwarfism called Munchkin joined the crew of Mayo Clinic service animals. Munchkin is 8 years old and has been a registered therapy animal for years. Now he and his human companion team up to provide support for Mayo Clinic patients. Munchkin is only permitted to visit a select few public lobbies around Mayo. His dwarfism also limits his ability to walk long distances, so he needs to remain close to a building entrance.

A **service dog** has been trained to perform specific tasks for someone who has a disability. For example, service dogs may be guiding people who are blind, alerting people who are deaf, pulling a wheelchair, protecting a person who is having a seizure or calming a person with post-traumatic stress disorder during an anxiety attack. They are also trained to do tasks such as opening doors and pushing buttons. Service animals are working animals, not pets. Service dogs live with the person they help and can accompany them in public areas such as mass transit, retail stores, restaurants and airplanes. They must be permitted in rental units or housing facilities, even if pets are not allowed.

A **facility dog** has traits of both a therapy dog and a service dog. It is a professionally trained dog that has learned skilled tasks to complement the work of a licensed clinical or professional provider and is accustomed to working longer hours in complex facilities. These dogs complete an extensive and specialized program, at the end of which they are certified by an Assistance Dogs International-accredited facility dog organization before they go on to help humans. Like service dogs, they can open doors and push buttons. But unlike service dogs, they don't live with or assist one person with disability. Instead, they work alongside their handlers providing support to many different people in hospital and other settings.

An **emotional support dog** is not a service dog, as it's not trained to assist people in the same way that service dogs do. Rather, an emotional support dog is considered a companion animal who eases anxiety, depression or loneliness. To be considered an emotional support dog, the dog must be prescribed by a mental health professional for a person with a diagnosed psychological or emotional disorder, such as anxiety, major depression or panic attacks. Emotional support dogs are considered pets. They don't have the same access as service dogs but may be considered a reasonable accommodation in specific situations.

OUR TAKE

Animal companionship offers many beloved advantages, but precautions apply. It's important to ensure safety and cleanliness during an interaction with an animal. Most hospitals and facilities that offer animal-assisted services have stringent rules to ensure that animal-handler teams are equipped to provide safe visits. The animals are clean, vaccinated, well trained and screened for appropriate personalities and behavior. The Centers for Disease Control and Prevention has yet to receive a report of infection from animal-assisted interventions. Note that when someone has an animal allergy or a suppressed immune system or simply doesn't enjoy interacting with animals, animal-assisted support isn't a good fit.

Aromatherapy

When walking through a blooming garden in the spring, you may have noticed that you like some scents more than others. You may have also noticed that certain scents affect you in specific ways. For example, lavender might make you feel more relaxed, while orange might leave you invigorated. You can ascribe these feelings to your personal preference in fragrances, but today we know that many scents can indeed have powerful effects on our mood and general well-being. Moreover, modern science knows exactly how scents work on your brain.

THE NOSE KNOWS

The reason your nose can detect smells is that fragrant substances give off specific molecules. As these molecules waft through the air and you inhale them, they bind to the smell-related, or olfactory, receptors in your nose. The receptors send chemical messages through the olfactory nerve to your brain. These messages talk to the brain's limbic system, which controls emotions and stores memories. The messages also stimulate the hypothalamus, which is responsible for hormones that affect your heart rate, hunger, body temperature and mood.

In response to a smell, your brain releases hormones such as:

- **Serotonin**, which plays a role in mood, sleep, digestion, nausea, wound healing, bone health and blood clotting.
- **Dopamine**, which regulates attention, learning, memory, mood and movement.
- **Endorphins**, which help relieve pain, reduce stress and improve mood.

Because these hormones help regulate many body functions, their release can help decrease anxiety or reduce your perception of pain. Aromatherapy draws on this science to gently and naturally aid the body and mind in dealing with physical and mental challenges. It's a holistic therapy — it supports mind, body and spirit.

HEALING SCENTS

Aromatherapy involves inhaling essential oils or applying them in a diluted form to the skin. Essential oils are highly concentrated and fragrant plant extracts, derived from flowers, leaves and stems. Some essential oils possess antimicrobial properties and can kill certain bacteria, fungi and viruses.

Because essential oils are so concentrated, use caution if applying directly to skin. Essential oils must be diluted in carrier or base oils, which are also made from plants but don't have a strong smell and don't give off the fragrant molecules. Base oils often contain antioxidants and essential fatty acids. They serve as vehicles to deliver essential oils while also nourishing your skin.

Our ancestors may not have understood the complex scientific underpinnings of aromatherapy and essential oils, but they surely knew their benefits — and harnessed them too. Many ancient cultures recognized the physical and mental benefits of scented ointments and oils. Inside Egyptian pyramids, archaeologists have found manuscripts describing the use of frankincense, myrrh and other herbs as medicine. In France, cave drawings dating back many thousands of years depict medicinal herbs. And a Neanderthal skeleton unearthed in modern-day Iraq was found buried with concentrated extracts of various plants, including yarrow, which today is used in aromatherapy and herbal medicine.

Using plants to improve physical and mental health has a rich global history. Greek physician Hippocrates, often described as the father of modern medicine, was known to say that "the key to good health rests on having a daily aromatic bath and scented massage." Greek physician and botanist Dioscorides listed many herbs and essential oils in use today in his medical book, including cardamom, cinnamon, myrrh, basil, fennel, frankincense, juniper, pine, rose, rosemary and thyme.

The modern term *aromatherapy* was coined in 1937 by French chemist René-Maurice Gattefossé. In 1910 he discovered the healing properties of lavender oil when he applied it to a burn on his hand caused by an explosion in his laboratory. That accident inspired him to analyze the chemical properties of essential oils and later to study how to use them to treat burns as well as wounds experienced by soldiers during World War I. During World War II, physicians did the same.

RELAXING SCENTS

Some common aromatherapy scents used for relaxation include:
- Lavender
- Jasmine
- Chamomile
- Bergamot
- Rose
- Clary sage
- Neroli
- Sandalwood
- Ylang-ylang
- Vanilla
- Lemon
- Ginger
- Geranium
- Tea tree
- Cedarwood

Today, aromatherapy is a fast-growing component of a holistic health approach. According to the National Center for Complementary and Integrative Health, Americans spend more than $30.2 billion annually on aromatherapy. Some estimates predict that by the year 2050, people worldwide will be spending $5 trillion on aromatherapy.

Recent studies illustrate how inhaling chemicals in essential oils work on the brain and body. For example, lavender and bergamot contain a compound called linalool that coaxes the brain to ease anxiety and depression. Cinnamon may decrease anxiety by inhibiting the release of pro-inflammatory cytokines, molecules that can cause harm if they get out of control. Sweet orange, rose and lavender can act as natural sedatives, as they reduce cortisol, the stress hormone. Rose also boosts serotonin while decreasing cortisol. Rosemary and clary sage can act as cognitive stimulants and memory enhancers. And a combination of various scents may produce a wide range of therapeutic effects.

There are many ways to inhale the oils' scents: You can use a nasal inhaler, a vapor diffuser, vapor balm, air spray or a cotton ball scented with a few drops of oil. Aromatherapy is often combined with a massage to aid relaxation and boost the overall wellness effect.

FINDING A QUALIFIED AROMATHERAPY PRACTITIONER
To find a certified aromatherapist in your area, consult the National Association for Holistic Aromatherapy (NAHA) website, *www.naha.org*. Another useful resource is the Alliance of International Aromatherapists, *www.alliance-aromatherapists.org*.

If you choose to use aromatherapy, keep your healthcare team informed in case you develop any kind of reactions or side effects.

Lavender and bergamot contain a chemical compound that, when inhaled, coaxes the brain to ease anxiety and depression. The scent of cinnamon may decrease anxiety, and the smells of sweet orange, rose and lavender can act as a natural sedatives. Rosemary and clary sage can act as brain stimulants and memory enhancers.

EXPERT INSIGHT
AROMATHERAPY AT MAYO CLINIC

Mayo Clinic began using aromatherapy over a decade ago, prompted by patients' interest. "I was working in cardiac surgery at the time, and we had many patients who were nauseated by some of the opioid medications," says Susanne M. Cutshall, a clinical nurse specialist who's been involved in setting up a number of integrative therapies at Mayo. "So we were trying to find other ways to provide comfort." Cutshall's team began using inhalers with four different oils often used for nausea.

Later, they introduced a disposable version of aromatherapy in the pediatric department — scented cotton balls in plastic baggies that children could sniff as needed.

Today, aromatherapy is used in many different areas of Mayo Clinic, including palliative care, says Cutshall. Aromatherapy is offered both as an inpatient and outpatient service. Essential oils commonly used at Mayo Clinic include lavender, mandarin, sweet orange, lemon, ginger, spearmint and frankincense. Lavender is a popular request.

"We don't recommend ingesting essential oils because they are chemicals from plants, so people could have a reaction to them. They could also interact with other medications people are taking," says Cutshall. "Our preferred method is by inhalation," adds Abbey K. Metzger, a Mayo Clinic nurse specializing in palliative care. "It is the safest and also the quickest because it goes straight to your olfactory system."

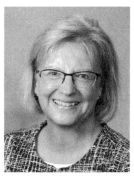

Susanne M. Cutshall, APRN, CNS, D.N.P.
Palliative Care

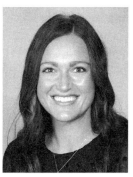

Abbey K. Metzger, D.N.P., R.N., CHPN
Palliative Care

WHAT THE RESEARCH SAYS

Aromatherapy is a holistic approach to health that can be used to improve general well-being. It also can be useful in the management of more specific conditions such as pain, nausea, anxiety, depression, stress and insomnia. Aromatherapy may be beneficial for preoperative anxiety and in cancer care and palliative care, and it can improve quality of life, particularly for people with chronic health conditions.

Pain

Aromatherapy may help ease pain. In one study, people who underwent coronary artery bypass surgery wore a lavender-scented gauze necklace for three days, with the fragrance replenished every 24 hours. Compared with the control group that wore unscented necklaces, these people experienced less postoperative pain. Researchers also found that aromatherapy with lavender oil may reduce pain and the number of painkillers given to children undergoing tonsillectomy. Another recent study recommended using aromatherapy as a pain relief option in the emergency departments of hospitals.

Anxiety

Anxiety is another area where aromatherapy appears helpful. One small study found that when burn patients inhaled rose essential oil, they were less anxious and slept better. A systematic review of multiple aromatherapy studies found that most reported a positive effect on anxiety levels compared with control groups, although the studies lacked proper details and precise descriptions of plant species and essential oil dosage.

Labor pain and anxiety

A data analysis examining aromatherapy use during labor found that it was effective at lessening pain in 11 out of 14 different trials. A systematic review of more than 30 studies also concluded that aromatherapy can reduce anxiety and pain during labor.

Sleep and fatigue

One study of 67 adults over 60 found that inhaling lavender essential oil boosted their levels of melatonin. Melatonin is a sleep hormone that typically decreases with age, a deficit that can contribute to insomnia.

A small study found that orange peel essential oil helped improve sleep in postpartum mothers but noted that larger studies are needed to recommend its use in health clinics.

An analysis of several studies found that aromatherapy can improve sleep quality and might be effective as a nondrug treatment for insomnia.

One study suggested that aromatherapy may relieve fatigue and sleep problems in people with irritable bowel syndrome, but the study design didn't allow researchers to determine whether the effects were real or due to placebo.

RISKS AND SAFETY CONCERNS

Although essential oils used in aromatherapy aren't regulated by the Food and Drug Administration, they're generally considered safe. But just because they're natural doesn't mean that they don't pose risks if used inappropriately. Pure essential oils are typically safe. Essential oils that are not pure may have added substances that might cause an allergic reaction. Inhaling too much may cause a headache.

When essential oils are applied to the skin, they may change skin composition, making it more prone to a reaction, skin irritation or burn. To avoid skin irritation, essential oils are often diluted with a carrier oil, such as coconut, jojoba or almond oil. It's a good idea to test an oil on a small patch of your skin first before applying it more broadly.

More research is needed to determine how essential oils might affect children and women who are pregnant or breastfeeding. Further investigation is also needed into how essential oils might interact with medications and other treatments.

OUR TAKE

Research on the effectiveness of aromatherapy continues, but there's a lack of well-designed studies, and more rigorous investigations are needed. It's important to find quality essential oils. When used appropriately, aromatherapy appears generally safe. It can help with relaxation, stress and anxiety reduction, and sleep. It can often bring a sense of comfort, and in some cases it can have a direct impact on specific symptoms. It also can act as a complement to pain medications. Many hospitals across the country are beginning to implement aromatherapy as a comfort measure.

Art therapy

At first, the young woman lying in the hospital bed wouldn't look at Lynn Borkenhagen, let alone talk to her. The patient had metastatic ovarian cancer and had come to Mayo Clinic looking for a miracle, but none was to be had. She had arrived at the hospital bright-eyed and hopeful, but over the course of three weeks she had retreated deep into herself. Staff caring for her had called on Borkenhagen, a palliative care nurse practitioner, for help.

Since the patient wouldn't speak, her husband filled the silence, telling Borkenhagen about his wife and their arranged marriage, which had blossomed into love. When he mentioned their 6-year-old daughter, the woman turned to Borkenhagen and finally spoke. "How will she remember how much I love her?" she asked.

"She was so concerned about her daughter," Borkenhagen says. "This woman knew she was dying. She needed a way to do legacy work for her daughter." So Borkenhagen reached out to Mayo's Arts at the Bedside program, part of Mayo's Center for Humanities in Medicine, which connects patients with writers, visual artists and musicians. A writer began coming to the woman's hospital room each day, working with her to capture the stories, memories and love that she wanted to leave behind for her family. "It was an epiphany," Borkenhagen says. "She started to become more herself again. She emotionally came to a better place. The experience was healing to the patient."

Jenna Whiting, a visual artist working with the same program, has seen that healing take place many times. Over the past several years, Whiting has experienced the difference that art — and the human connection that accompanies it — can make to people facing difficult circumstances. A couple of days a week, Whiting loads up a large canvas bag with various art mediums and makes visits to patients throughout Mayo Clinic hospitals. "I bring different materials depending on which unit I'm going to visit," she says.

For example, decorating plain onesies and crafting personalized nursery artwork are popular with expectant mothers who are hospitalized. In palliative care and oncology areas, it's often watercolor pencils, canvas painting or greeting cards. "I pop into patient rooms, explain what the program is all about and ask if they're interested in creating something," she says. If the answer is yes, Whiting pulls out her materials and engages the patient in a type of care that has nothing to do with tests or treatments. "I'm not there to poke or do checks on the patient. I am simply

86   Mayo Clinic Guide to Holistic Health

there to spend time with them and connect creatively and through conversations, getting to know them outside of their diagnosis," Whiting says.

This connection serves as a good reminder of what — or rather, *who* — healthcare is all about. "We aren't treating a disease; we're treating a person," Borkenhagen says. "It's so important for providers to turn away from the computers and be present with patients. To open their hearts to patients and hear their stories. People are more than just their diseases. We need to explore all avenues for healing our patients, and the arts are another avenue of healing."

ART AND HEALING

The idea of using art to help with difficult health moments isn't new. For thousands of years, people have been using arts such as singing, painting and dancing for healing purposes. Around the 1940s, healthcare professionals noticed that people with mental illness would express themselves through art. This observation inspired the use of creative arts therapy as a healing technique for conditions including anxiety, depression, schizophrenia and dementia.

You might use art to support your own well-being without even thinking about it. Maybe you doodle when you feel stressed or you enjoy playing an instrument at the end of a long day. Artistic expression and appreciation are not only enjoyable but also have the potential to benefit your health.

Today, art is used to help treat specific conditions, promote overall well-being and even help prevent diseases. Self-expression through art therapy can help people cope with mood disorders and other mental and emotional issues. Art therapy involves the use of drawing, painting, sculpture and other art forms to allow expression and organization of your inner thoughts and emotions when talking about them is difficult. Creative arts therapy can help process emotions, enhance focus, facilitate communication and increase self-esteem.

The creation of art itself, or the interpretation of an art piece, is thought to be therapeutic. The focus is not on the final product; it is about healing through the process of making or experiencing art.

Art therapy is practiced in a wide variety of settings, including hospitals, psychiatric and rehabilitation facilities, wellness centers, schools, crisis centers, senior communities, private practices and other clinical and community settings, and in both individual and group sessions.

Your brain on art

Research finds that the process of making art has a physical effect on the body and mind. In particular, it affects the brain's ability to change and adapt, a characteristic called neuroplasticity — a feature that can help people recover from traumatic brain injuries or stroke.

Evidence suggests that art enhances brain function by impacting brain wave patterns, emotional centers and the nervous system. These benefits don't just come from making art; they also occur from experiencing art. Observing art can stimulate the creation of new neural pathways and ways of thinking.

Whether it's part of a creative arts therapy exercise or something you experience in your everyday life, art can help you:

- **Lower stress** Creating art can reduce the levels of the stress hormone cortisol and increase the levels of serotonin — the feel-good hormone. This happens for those who identify as artists and those who don't, so no matter your skill level, everyone can benefit from making art.
- **Focus** Art allows people to enter a "flow state" — that feeling that develops when you're "in the zone" and lose your sense of self and time. Making art also activates a variety of brain networks, including a relaxed reflective state, focused attention and pleasure.
- **Process emotions** Art allows you to express feelings and memories in ways other than words. Making art can be a cathartic experience for those dealing with distress and can provide a sense of relief.
- **Imagine a more hopeful future** Human brains tend to predict the future based on what has happened in the recent past. Creating art prompts you to make decisions and interpret images, figuring out their meaning. That frame of mind can help you face the future, as well as imagine a better, more hopeful way ahead for yourself.
- **Experience positive emotions and pleasure** Research shows that when people view art they consider beautiful, they experience increased blood flow to the part of the brain associated with pleasure.

How art therapy is used

Music, dance, writing, storytelling, collage-making and painting can all be used in creative arts therapy. Creative arts therapists draw upon their training to meet the needs and interests of patients. The success of art

 Research has identified a range of physical and mental health benefits of art and art therapy.

therapy is measured not by the quality of the art produced in a session but by the healing that can happen during the process of making art. In healthcare settings, art therapy is usually used in two ways.

- **Arts in health**, which can include artists trained to help patients have positive creative experiences. It can be practiced in hospitals and healthcare facilities. This might also include art on the walls, musical performances in the lobby and healing gardens.
- **Creative arts therapies**, which include a licensed professional engaging a patient in arts to address a specific condition or meet a health goal. Therapy can be delivered through visual art, dance, music, poetry or drama, and there are corresponding licenses for each type of art specialization.

WHAT THE RESEARCH SAYS
Research has identified a range of physical and mental health benefits of art and art therapy.

Brain-related disorders
A 2014 review of research studies focused on the use of art therapy for Alzheimer's disease. The authors of the review concluded that art therapy engages attention, provides pleasure and improves neuropsychiatric symptoms, social behavior and self-esteem in people who have Alzheimer's disease.

Several literature reviews found that art therapy can be a useful complementary treatment for mood disorders such as anxiety or depression and mental disorders such as schizophrenia and autism.

Cancer and related treatment
Several studies found that art therapy improved anxiety, depression and pain symptoms in people with cancer, and it decreased their fatigue and improved their overall quality of life. In one study, patients reported increased feelings of hope after 4 out of 5 therapy sessions.

OUR TAKE
There's preliminary evidence that both making art and viewing art influence emotions and the brain's neuroplasticity in a positive way. Research finds that art enhances brain function by affecting brain wave patterns, emotions and the nervous system. Art also helps reduce stress, improve focus and foster positive thoughts and optimism. There's little harm in experimenting with art therapy, and it may provide a real benefit.

Biofeedback

Biofeedback is a mind-body technique, assisted by technology, in which you learn to consciously modify your body's responses to different triggers. Doing so can improve your physical, mental, emotional and spiritual health. It's like taking charge of your body rather than your body controlling you.

When you're in pain or under stress, your body functions change. Your heart rate may increase, you may breathe faster and your muscles may tighten up. Biofeedback therapy uses sensors attached to your skin to measure these responses and relay them back to you via graphs or charts. With this knowledge, you make slight adjustments to your body, such as relaxing certain muscles to help relieve pain or reduce tension, or slowing your heart rate and breathing to help you feel calmer. This can improve a health problem or make daily activities easier. Common disorders treated by biofeedback include hypertension, anxiety and medical conditions exacerbated by stress.

Biofeedback is often conducted while you're attached to a machine in a health professional's office. But it also can be done using wearable devices at a medical center or, increasingly, at home.

Just as looking into a mirror allows you to see and change your facial expressions, biofeedback allows you to see "inside" your body, while a trained practitioner guides you on how to shift your physical responses in a healthy direction. As a result, you learn to voluntarily control what you once thought were involuntary body processes. For example, you may learn to decrease your physiological stress response by regulating some of your body's functions such as heart rate, breathing and muscle tightness. Over time you can learn to self-regulate without looking at the feedback screen, so you can do this anywhere.

WHY IT'S DONE
Biofeedback, also called biofeedback training, appeals to people for a variety of reasons, including:
- There's no surgery or discomfort involved — it's a noninvasive treatment.
- It might reduce or eliminate the need for medicines.
- It might make medicines work better.
- It might help when medicines can't be used, such as during pregnancy, or when they are not effective.
- It helps people feel more in control of their health.

90   Mayo Clinic Guide to Holistic Health

Biofeedback is most commonly used for managing chronic symptoms due to anxiety or pain, but it can be used for many conditions (see "What the research says" on page 96).

TYPES OF BIOFEEDBACK

Your therapist might use different kinds of biofeedback depending on your health problems and goals. Biofeedback types include:

- **Breathing** During breathing biofeedback, bands are placed around your stomach and chest. Sensors on the bands check your breathing rate and patterns. Learning to adjust your breathing can help you feel better.
- **Brain waves** During this type of biofeedback, an electroencephalograph (EEG) uses scalp pads to monitor your brain waves. There are certain brain waves that show different mental states, such as relaxation, wakefulness and sleep. With biofeedback training, you can see a change in the brain waves that improve your health.
- **Heart rate** In this type of biofeedback, pads are placed on your chest, lower trunk or wrists. These pads are connected to an electrocardiogram (ECG), which measures your heart rate and how your heart rate changes. A sensor also can be placed on your finger to measure your heart rate. When you're relaxed, your heart rate tends to decrease.
- **Muscle activity** A machine called an electromyograph (EMG) uses sensors to measure muscle tightening. This helps make you aware of muscle tension so you can take steps to relax tight muscles.
- **Sweat gland activity** Pads attached to your fingers, palm or wrist measure the activity of the sweat glands. The amount of perspiration on your skin can help indicate nervousness.
- **Temperature** Pads attached to your fingers or feet measure blood flow to your skin. Because your temperature often drops when you're under stress, a low temperature reading can prompt you to start relaxing. As you become calmer, your fingers and toes may become warmer.

WHAT YOU CAN EXPECT DURING THE TREATMENT

During biofeedback, a therapist connects electrical pads or sensors to different parts of your body. These pads might be used to:

- Monitor your brain waves.
- Check the temperature of your skin.
- Measure muscle tightness.
- Monitor your heart rate.
- Monitor your breathing rate and patterns.

The pads send information to a nearby screen. The therapist uses that information and makes suggestions to help you control your body's responses. For example, if the pads sense tight muscles that may be causing headaches, you then learn how to relax those muscles.

A typical biofeedback treatment lasts 30 to 60 minutes. How many treatments you have and how long they last depend on your health problem and how quickly you learn to control your body's responses. The goal of biofeedback is to learn to sense and then control the responses on your own without a machine or sensors.

HOW TO FIND A QUALIFIED PRACTITIONER

To find a person who teaches biofeedback, ask your healthcare team to recommend someone who has experience treating your problem. Many

---

BIOFEEDBACK AT HOME

Most people receive biofeedback training in physical therapy clinics, medical centers or hospitals. But a growing number of biofeedback machines and programs are being marketed for home use. The following are examples of biofeedback home devices.

Interactive computer programs or mobile devices
Changes in your heart rate and skin are measured with pads attached to your fingers or your ear. The measuring pads plug into your computer. Using computer pictures and cues, the machines help you manage nervousness by guiding you to modify your breathing, relax your muscles and think positively about your ability to deal with stress. Studies show that these types of machines might help you deal with stress and make you calmer.

Wearable devices
One type of biofeedback treatment involves wearing a headband that tracks your brain activity while you meditate. It uses sounds to let you know when your mind is calm and when it's active. Information from your meditation sessions is stored on your computer or mobile device so you can track your progress over time.

Another type is a measuring pad placed on your waist to monitor your breathing patterns using a downloadable app. The app can let biofeedback experts are licensed in another area of healthcare, as well, such as psychology, nursing or physical therapy. Search for a qualified biofeedback practitioner at *www.bcia.org/consumers-find-a-practitioner*.

State laws regulating biofeedback teaching vary. Some biofeedback experts choose to become certified to show their extra training and experience in the practice. The Biofeedback Certification Institute of America offers various levels of certification. Before starting treatment, consider asking the biofeedback expert a few questions, such as:

- Are you licensed, certified or registered?
- What is your training and experience?
- Do you have experience teaching biofeedback for my problem?
- How many biofeedback treatments do you think I'll need?
- What's the cost and is it covered by my health insurance?
- Can you give me a list of references?

you know if your breathing rate accelerates and give you breathing activities to restore calm.

The FDA has approved a biofeedback machine, Resperate, for decreasing stress and lowering blood pressure. The portable electronic machine helps you practice slow, deep breathing. Chest sensors measure your breathing rate, then send the real-time information to a small device worn on a belt. The device creates a melody for you to listen to and synchronize your breathing with. The melody is designed to help you slow your breathing with long exhalations.

Resperate is intended to be used at least 15 minutes a day, 3 or 4 days a week. Within a few weeks, the device-guided slow breathing exercises may help lower both the top (systolic) and bottom (diastolic) numbers in a blood pressure reading.

Choose wisely

Keep in mind that the Food and Drug Administration (FDA) doesn't regulate all biofeedback machines made for home use. Before trying biofeedback therapy at home, talk with your healthcare team about different machines so you can find the best fit. Also, be aware that some items might be falsely sold as biofeedback machines, and some people who offer biofeedback may not be certified or have enough training to help you.

EXPERT INSIGHT
BIOFEEDBACK AT MAYO CLINIC

Mayo Clinic uses biofeedback techniques to benefit more than 800 people a year. Experts from a variety of disciplines work with biofeedback specialists to coordinate a holistic, more comprehensive approach to treatment.

Presently there is a biofeedback revolution going on, states Ivana T. Croghan, Ph.D., a researcher at Mayo Clinic. Over the past few years, she's observed how biofeedback technologies have made a quantum leap, offering so much more data than what they did before. This is largely due to the advent of wearable technology.

In the recent past, people thought of biofeedback equipment as large machines to which patients were hooked up in clinical settings. Patients would work through a session and gain knowledge, but then go home where they wouldn't be able to use any of the equipment. Wearable technologies have changed that. Now people may use biofeedback in the comfort of their own homes, thanks to a wide range of wearable tech devices and smartphone apps.

These wearable devices, often referred to as wearables, can read and measure a person's temperature, breathing rate, oxygen levels, heart rate and even brainwave activity. The wearables then transfer the information to the apps. "We're actually working with several new devices currently," says Dr. Croghan. "These devices can communicate with accompanying apps and transfer relevant information."

One of Dr. Croghan's studies involves a biofeedback device that guides a person into a meditative state. "This device uses biofeedback to recognize when you are in a meditative state, and with the assistance of the accompanying app, helps you maintain that meditative state for at least three minutes," she says. "In our research, we have found that this can reduce stress and anxiety."

Dr. Croghan's team investigated several such novel biofeedback devices, particularly during the pandemic when stress among healthcare professionals was extremely high. For example, they studied BreatherFit, a respiratory muscle-training device used by Mayo Clinic staff in the Stress Resilience Program, and saw results effective enough to recommend it as an option for reducing stress. Another product, a wearable brain-sensing device called MUSE-S, provided guided meditation sessions. Participating Mayo Clinic physicians wore it as a headband to listen to the recorded meditation sessions. Dr. Croghan's team found that 3 to 10 minutes of this practice during work hours helped the physicians better cope with stress. Another study investigated a virtual reality device, Reulay Oculus, with similar positive outcomes (see page 216 for more on virtual reality).

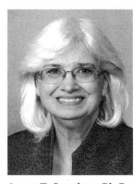

Ivana T. Croghan, Ph.D.
General Internal Medicine

These biofeedback devices can help you get into a meditative state when taking your mind off things is difficult, Dr. Croghan says. "How many times do people tell you to 'just meditate, do yoga,' and you say to yourself, 'OK, but I can't clear my mind'? You try to do it yourself, and it's not effective. But when you utilize these biofeedback systems, they are instructing you step by step on how to utilize them. The more you listen, and the more you practice with them, the more you improve. Eventually you reach the point where you no longer need the app or the device. You can do it yourself."

Different devices work for different people, states Dr. Croghan. For some, audio instructions are sufficient to ease into them into the meditative state. Others prefer the visual settings of virtual reality.

"The version we have right now has several different kinds of virtual realities," Dr. Croghan says. "For example, one of them is just taking a walk through the woods. Another one is walking on the beach. Yet another one is walking among cherry blossoms in Japan. All of them can guide you into a designated state — take a look around, breathe deep, hear the sound of the stream — those types of things which can calm you down. Many prior participants found the visualization to be extremely beneficial."

WHAT THE RESEARCH SAYS

Biofeedback is useful for treating many physical and mental health conditions. Studies indicate it has the potential to improve symptoms of asthma, Raynaud's disease, irritable bowel syndrome, constipation, incontinence, chronic pain, headache, anxiety, stress, high blood pressure, stroke and others. Research into its effectiveness in these and other areas is ongoing.

Stress and anxiety

One Mayo Clinic study found that computer sessions using biofeedback to reinforce training devices significantly reduced stress and anxiety in hospital personnel during the pandemic. Three other Mayo Clinic studies found that wearable biofeedback devices — such as BreatherFit, MUSE-S and Reulay Oculus — similarly alleviated stress, increased resilience and improved thinking and memory processes in healthcare personnel.

Headache

One study investigated using a biofeedback app for migraine and found it to be a useful intervention.

Asthma

Other research indicates biofeedback may be a promising protective, complementary approach that can help reduce impairment of lung function due to psychological stress.

Chronic pain

A small study found biofeedback can help reduce the perception of pain in people with chronic low back pain, as well as reduce stress. The study also noted biofeedback's positive effects on self-awareness and sleep.

Studies indicate biofeedback has the potential to improve symptoms of asthma, Raynaud's disease, irritable bowel syndrome, constipation, incontinence, chronic pain, headache, anxiety, stress, high blood pressure, stroke and others.

Arthritis

According to one research effort, biofeedback increased the efficiency of the rehabilitation process in people with rheumatoid arthritis and helped boost their levels of self-control.

RISKS AND SAFETY CONCERNS

Biofeedback is generally safe. Almost anyone can use it, and it can be used for any age group. In a few rare cases, it might not work well. Biofeedback machines might not work on people with certain medical problems, such as heartbeat issues or some skin diseases. If you have a medical condition, it's helpful to talk with your healthcare team before trying biofeedback.

OUR TAKE

Biofeedback is, for the most part, safe, widely used and accepted, and practiced in many medical centers. With a qualified therapist and proper instruction and supervision, biofeedback may be useful as part of a comprehensive and holistic treatment plan, as long as the person is actively participating in the learning process.

Not all insurance companies pay for biofeedback, so be sure to find out whether your insurance provider does.

A growing number of wearable devices can now provide quality biofeedback on how your body is responding to meditation instructions or calming scenery, so they can be helpful too. Some biofeedback wearables can be expensive, so choose wisely and consult with your healthcare team if you have questions.

Cannabis and cannabinoids

Cannabis is a plant that's long been used for both medicinal and recreational purposes. Some people know it as hemp, others as marijuana. Many people believe it helps them cope with anxiety, insomnia, nausea and other common ailments. Health professionals aren't so sure.

The history of cannabis is rife with twists and turns (see opposite page). After being vilified in the last century, it has reemerged as a potential therapeutic. Even though the U.S. federal government still considers it illegal, nearly three-quarters of states in the U.S. have set up systems over the last three decades to provide access to therapeutic cannabis. A smaller number of states also have legalized cannabis for recreational use. The list of conditions that states have approved for treatment is varied and expansive.

CANNABIS, CANNABINOIDS, MARIJUANA, HEMP, CBD, THC — WHAT'S THE DIFFERENCE?

People often use the words *cannabis* and *marijuana* interchangeably, but they don't mean exactly the same thing.

- The word *cannabis* refers to all products derived from the plant. The cannabis plant contains about 540 chemical substances.
- The word *marijuana* refers to parts of or products from the plant that contain substantial amounts of tetrahydrocannabinol or THC, the substance that's primarily responsible for the effects of marijuana on a person's mental state — the so-called high.
- Cannabinoids are a group of substances found in the cannabis plant. The main cannabinoids are THC and cannabidiol or CBD. Unlike THC, CBD does not impair a person's mental state and doesn't produce a high. Besides THC and CBD, there are more than 100 other cannabinoids.
- Marijuana and hemp are essentially two different strains of the same plant. THC and CBD are the most common cannabinoids found in marijuana and hemp. The difference is that hemp generally contains low amounts of THC and high amounts of CBD, while marijuana generally contains high amounts of THC and low amounts of CBD. Under U.S. law, cannabis plants containing 0.3% or less of THC are classified as hemp, and cannabis plants containing more than 0.3% of THC are classified as marijuana.
- Synthetic cannabinoids or synthetic marijuana are lab-made substances that are chemically similar to compounds found in cannabis

98   Mayo Clinic Guide to Holistic Health

? DID YOU KNOW?

The oldest known written record that mentions cannabis use dates to the Chinese emperor Shen Nung, in 2727 B.C.E. However, archaeologists have found evidence that humans have used cannabis a lot longer than that — for nearly 12,000 years. As a plant, called hemp, cannabis was extremely useful, providing fibers for ropes and nets, food, and seeds for oil. Cannabis was widely used in ancient societies, often described by a similar-sounding name. In Latin it was *cannabis,* in Arabic *qunnab,* in Italian *canapa,* in Russian *konoplja* and in Georgian *kanap'is.*

Our ancestors realized the plant's euphoria-inducing properties early on. According to Indian mythology, the god Shiva supposedly favored cannabis, which was used as an agent for mystic inspiration in religious ceremonies. It also was used in traditional Ayurvedic medicine to reduce pain, anxiety and nausea; relax muscles; and improve appetite and sleep, in addition to producing a feeling of ecstasy. The Egyptians applied cannabis topically to treat inflammation, according to papyrus records from 1500 B.C.E. Along the same lines, Greek physician Dioscorides wrote in his book *De Materia Medica* that using boiled root of cannabis could decrease inflammation.

Irish physician William O'Shaughnessy Brooke introduced cannabis to Europe in the 1800s. He used it as medicine to relieve spasms in cases of tetanus, cholera and convulsive disorders. Later, Western medics of the 19th and early 20th centuries used cannabis for pain. Queen Victoria took it for painful menses, while Empress Elisabeth (Sissi) of Austria used it for cough and possibly also to stimulate appetite. An 1862 issue of *Vanity Fair* advertised hashish candy — another cannabis product — for nervousness and melancholy as well as "a pleasurable and harmless stimulant." The advertisement added that "under its influence all classes seem to gather new inspiration and energy."

During the 20th century, cannabis gradually fell out of favor, viewed as a narcotic for its mind-altering qualities. Between 1914 and 1925, 26 U.S. states passed laws prohibiting its use. In 1937, Congress passed the Marijuana Tax Act, essentially criminalizing its use. Decades later, in 1970, Congress passed the Comprehensive Drug Abuse Prevention and Control Act, which disallowed marijuana use in medical practice. It would take nearly 50 years to change that view.

plants. Yet, because they are made in the lab, they can be very different from the plant-based compounds. The U.S. Food and Drug Administration has approved some synthetic versions.

THE ENDOCANNABINOID SYSTEM OF THE HUMAN BODY
The human body produces its own version of chemicals very similar to THC. These substances are called endocannabinoids, the prefix *endo-* meaning "internal" or "internally produced." Scientists found that from an evolutionary perspective, the appearance of endocannabinoids in animals predates the appearance of the plant by about 600 million years.

Endocannabinoids are produced by various parts of the body, including the brain, muscles, immune system and fatty tissue. Research shows that endocannabinoids are critical for many body functions that regulate human health, such as inflammation and other immune functions.

THE CANNABIS RENAISSANCE
In 2018, the U.S. Congress passed and signed into law the Agriculture Improvement Act. This law removed hemp from the federal Controlled Substances Act, effectively legalizing CBD that comes from hemp. Then, in 2022, Congress signed the Medical Marijuana and Cannabidiol Research Expansion Act to allow cannabis research for medical purposes. Many states have legalized cannabis for medical as well as recreational use.

People often use the words *cannabis* and *marijuana* interchangeably, but they don't mean the same thing.
› The word *cannabis* refers to all products derived from the plant.
› The word *marijuana* refers to parts of or products from the plant that contain substantial amounts of tetrahydrocannabinol or THC, the substance that's primarily responsible for the so-called high.
› Cannabinoids are a group of substances found in the cannabis plant.

In recent years, the FDA approved one cannabis-derived drug and three synthetic cannabis-type drugs for specific, hard-to-treat conditions.
- Epidiolex, which contains a purified form of CBD, is approved for the treatment of seizures associated with Lennox-Gastaut syndrome or Dravet syndrome. Epidiolex does not alter a person's mental state.
- Marinol and Syndros are two synthetic THC-containing drugs approved for chemotherapy-related nausea as well as for anorexia and appetite loss in AIDS patients. Marinol and Syndros can result in a high.
- Cesamet, also a synthetic drug that contains a THC-like compound, is approved for chemotherapy-related nausea.

These approved drugs are available only with a prescription from a licensed healthcare professional, the agency notes. Outside of these specific conditions, medical use of cannabis is still considered illegal at the federal level. Up to now, the FDA has not approved any other cannabis, cannabis-derived or CBD products sold without a prescription.

WHAT THE RESEARCH SAYS
So far cannabinoids have been consistently effective only for specific types of epilepsy, chemotherapy-related nausea and anorexia and appetite loss in AIDS patients, which is why the FDA approved cannabinoids for use in these conditions.

Several recent studies investigated the use of cannabinoids for various other conditions, including pain, anxiety, sleep problems, post-traumatic stress disorder, multiple sclerosis, inflammatory bowel disease, irritable bowel syndrome and even glaucoma. But many produced insufficient evidence or inconsistent results.

Pain
A 2017 review looked at studies in which cannabinoids were administered to people along with opioids to treat pain, with the goal of reducing opioid use. There were nine studies (750 total participants), of which three (642 participants) used a high-quality study design, meaning participants were randomly assigned to receive cannabinoids or a placebo. The results were inconsistent, and none of the high-quality studies indicated that cannabinoids could lead to decreased opioid use.

Anxiety
There's some evidence that cannabinoids can reduce anxiety. One study of 24 people with social anxiety disorder found that they had less anxiety in a simulated public speaking test after taking CBD than after taking a placebo. Other studies have suggested that cannabinoids may be helpful

for anxiety in people with chronic pain, but the study participants did not necessarily have anxiety disorders. A meta-analysis of several studies suggested that CBD indeed decreased anxiety in some people but wasn't as efficient in improving sleep.

Multiple sclerosis
Several small studies used the FDA-approved cannabinoids for treatment in multiple sclerosis. Some found small improvements in spasticity, pain and bladder problems as reported by the participants, while others did not.

Post-traumatic stress disorder
In a very small study of 10 people, cannabinoids provided a significant relief for military personnel with nightmares related to post-traumatic stress disorder, indicating promise as a potential therapeutic. However, other studies were less conclusive.

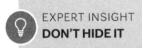

EXPERT INSIGHT
DON'T HIDE IT

Ann Vincent, M.D., an internist at Mayo Clinic, became interested in studying cannabis because of her patients. They would tell her that cannabis helped them with conditions such as arthritis, nerve pain and insomnia. Dr. Vincent appreciates that her patients talk with her about their use of cannabis. "Now that cannabis is available over the counter just like multivitamins, it's very important to discuss it," Dr. Vincent says.

Since cannabis is illegal at the federal level, physicians still can't prescribe or recommend cannabis to their patients, with the exception of FDA-approved cannabis medications for indications such as Dravet syndrome (see page 101). In states where cannabis is approved for certain medical conditions, patients can work with their state cannabis program to obtain a cannabis card for medical conditions approved by the state cannabis program.

Since cannabinoids can interact with many commonly prescribed medications, it's essential for patients to discuss cannabis use with their healthcare teams. Additionally, cannabis can impact people differently based on their genetic makeup. A certain percentage of

RISKS AND SAFETY CONCERNS

There are many ways of using cannabis, including smoking, vaping, consuming edibles or sublingual drops, or using topical forms applied to the skin. Research data to show which method is the safest is not currently available. But topical formats are likely to have the fewest undesirable effects — and here's why. Cannabinoids taken by mouth have the potential to interact with other medications in your system — and that can cause toxicity, either from the cannabis or from the other medications. Inhaling cannabinoids can rapidly increase their concentration in your blood, which can cause side effects. Meanwhile, applying them to skin doesn't carry the risk of these problems, so that method is the least likely to have harmful effects.

Cannabis and cannabinoids are not without risks. There are many concerns associated with the use of both.
- The use of cannabis has been linked to an increased risk of motor vehicle crashes.

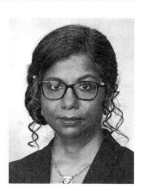

Ann Vincent, M.D.
General Internal Medicine

people may have atypical genetic variants that cause them to metabolize cannabis differently than people without these genetic variants. As a result, they may have higher or lower levels of cannabinoids in their systems than people without the variants, and may experience harmful effects. Currently there isn't enough data to fully understand the differences or set the doses correctly for each person.

If you are thinking of using cannabis, don't be afraid to discuss it with your healthcare team, Dr. Vincent says. And even though physicians can't legally recommend cannabis, they can talk to their patients about it and offer advice. "The attitude towards cannabis is now a little bit more relaxed. Because it can interact with medications it is important to discuss this aspect. Let's have a discussion. Let's get you some resources. Let's see if it's appropriate."

- Smoking cannabis during pregnancy has been linked to lower birth weight.
- Some people who use cannabis develop cannabis use disorder, which produces symptoms such as cravings, withdrawal, lack of control and negative effects on personal and professional responsibilities.
- Adolescents using cannabis are 4 to 7 times more likely than adults to develop cannabis use disorder.
- Cannabis use has been associated with an increased risk of falling among older adults.
- The use of cannabis, especially frequent use, has been linked to a higher risk of developing schizophrenia or other psychoses (severe mental illnesses) in people who are predisposed to these illnesses.
- Marijuana may cause a head rush or dizziness on standing up, possibly raising the risk of danger from fainting and falls.
- The FDA has warned the public not to use vaping products that contain THC. Products of this type have been implicated in many of the reported cases of serious lung injuries linked to vaping.
- There have been many reports of unintentional consumption of cannabis or its products by children, leading to illnesses severe enough to require emergency room treatment or hospitalization. Among a group of children and adults who became ill after accidental exposure to candies containing THC, the children generally had more severe symptoms than the adults and needed to stay in the hospital longer.
- There have been reports of contamination of cannabis and cannabinoid products with harmful microorganisms, pesticides and other substances.
- Some cannabis and cannabinoid products contain amounts of cannabinoids that differ substantially from what's stated on their labels.
- Some long-term users of high doses of cannabis have developed a condition involving recurrent severe vomiting. Even though cannabis can relieve nausea induced by chemotherapy, its prolonged use can result in recurrent nausea, vomiting and abdominal pain. Mayo Clinic researchers documented nearly 100 such cases in a study.

CBD also can have its own side effects. Unlike Epidiolex, the purified CBD product sold as an FDA-approved prescription drug, over-the-counter CBD products may contain more or less CBD than stated on their labels, and because of less rigorous regulatory oversight than what's required for prescription drugs, they also may contain contaminants, such as THC.

Although it does not produce a high, CBD may cause a drop in alertness, changes in mood, decreased appetite and gastrointestinal symptoms such as diarrhea. CBD may produce psychotic effects or cognitive

Cannabinoids are effective for a small number of conditions, such as epilepsy, nausea and loss of appetite.

impairment in people who also regularly use THC. In addition, CBD use has been associated with liver injury, male reproductive harm and interactions with other drugs. Some side effects, such as diarrhea, sleepiness, abnormalities on tests of liver function and drug interactions, appear to be due to CBD itself rather than contaminants in CBD products; these effects were observed in some of the people who participated in studies of Epidiolex before its approval as a drug.

OUR TAKE

Cannabinoids have proved to be helpful for a small number of hard-to-treat conditions. They are commonly available as over-the-counter medications in many states, but because these preparations are not regulated by the FDA, they may contain impurities and doses may vary from product to product. Additionally, cannabinoids affect each person differently and may interact with other medications. If you choose to use them, be sure to discuss your plans with your healthcare team and proceed with caution.

Cryotherapy

Imagine this: You walk into something that looks like a sauna, but instead of feeling a pleasant relaxing warmth, the chamber greets you with a freezing blast that would make an arctic wind feel like a spring breeze. That's not an overstatement, because the air being blown at you has been cooled to minus-148 degrees F or below.

Why would anyone subject themselves to such a chilling experience? While it may not sound very pleasant, the concept is similar to applying ice to an injury. Ice is used to prevent or decrease inflammatory processes that cause swelling, so the idea is that exposing the whole body to a blast of frigid air might do the same. Evidence is still lacking on the safety and effectiveness of more engineered forms of extreme cold treatment such as cryotherapy chambers. But some people are already using them and have been for a while, whether in professional athletic facilities, wellness resorts or local spas.

HOW DOES IT WORK?

Using cold to boost health isn't exactly a novel idea. Early cultures used cold as a traditional method of pain relief. In ancient Greece, Persia and Rome, chilly remedies such as snow, ice-and-water mixtures and cold water were used to treat a wide range of diseases. Ice water plunging remains a common tradition in many northern countries. And until about 1980, some psychiatric patients in the United States were wrapped in cold, wet sheets; the practice seemed to calm down agitated patients and stimulate those who were apathetic. The idea behind these seemingly unpleasant interventions was that it caused physiological reactions that boosted the immune system and jump-started physical activity.

Nowadays wet sheets have been replaced by cryotherapy chambers, in which cooling is done by a blast of frigid air. During these exposures, you wear minimal clothing, gloves, a woolen headband covering the ears, a nose and mouth mask, and dry shoes and socks to reduce the risk of cold-related injury. The blasts blow over fast — they last only 2 to 3 minutes. Admittedly, they probably feel far more jarring than wet sheets, but research finds that this extreme therapy is not entirely without scientific evidence and may offer some benefits.

Many professional athletes have been using whole-body cryotherapy for some time, often in the form of ice baths or plunges. Its popularity in sports stems from the belief that cryotherapy can help lower inflammation and soothe sore muscles — just like an ice pack, albeit with a greater chilling punch.

WHAT THE RESEARCH SAYS

Research into cryotherapy is still in its infancy. So far, cryotherapy has been used in sports medicine and also with some success in the treatment of inflammatory conditions such as rheumatoid arthritis and multiple sclerosis. It seems to have other potential uses as well.

Rheumatoid arthritis

Several studies found that whole-body cryotherapy at temperatures below minus-148 degrees F for a very short duration of time — about 2 to 3 minutes — helped decrease pain related to rheumatoid arthritis.

One study found that cryotherapy improved mobility and reduced the intensity of pain in people with rheumatoid arthritis, and that the positive effect lasted at least three months afterward. Several studies also recorded a measurable decrease in specific inflammatory markers after the therapy, showing that the improvement wasn't just based on the perception of the participant but was backed by the body's changing biology.

A systematic review of the literature suggested that cryotherapy for people with arthritis may have even larger effects. Those with rheumatoid arthritis often have difficulty exercising due to pain, for example, which affects their overall well-being, including heart health. The review suggested that cryotherapy can be an innovative strategy to improve a person's exercise capacity, thus reducing cardiovascular risk and boosting overall wellness.

Multiple sclerosis

Less research has been done on cryotherapy for multiple sclerosis, but one small study found that it had some measurable antioxidant benefits, which are helpful in fighting neurodegenerative disease.

Chronic low back pain

Another small study found whole-body cryotherapy to be effective for treating chronic low back pain. Cryotherapy decreased measurable inflammatory markers and boosted anti-inflammatory markers.

Heart health

Cryotherapy may boost the body's antioxidant response and exercise capacity. Early studies of whole-body cryotherapy concluded that it's generally safe and doesn't negatively affect cardiac or immunological health. Another recent systematic review found that cryotherapy may lower levels of cholesterol and triglycerides.

Mental health
Preliminary evidence suggests that whole-body cryotherapy may be useful as an add-on intervention for mental health problems, especially for symptoms of depression. Research has also found that cryotherapy may enhance quality of sleep and decrease tiredness.

Weight loss
A very recent study incorporated whole-body cryotherapy into a more traditional treatment plan for people with obesity who also experienced various post-COVID conditions, such as pain, poor sleep and muscle fatigue. In addition to exercising and eating a healthy diet, study participants went through cryotherapy. After four weeks, participants lost weight, became leaner and had lower cholesterol and inflammation markers than at the beginning of the study.

RISKS AND SAFETY CONCERNS
Cryotherapy is not for everybody. It's an intense and acute form of intervention. While it may work for some, others may not be able to tolerate it. Notably, humans have a much lower capacity to adapt to prolonged exposure to cold compared with prolonged exposure to heat. Even if cryotherapy sessions are very short, they still may be too extreme for some people. Acute exposure to a cold environment, either air or water, causes a stress reaction, as well as a temporary jump in blood pressure. That's because cold causes the blood vessels to temporarily constrict, which in turn results in higher pressure. There also may be other negative effects that aren't known yet.

OUR TAKE
Cryotherapy as a form of treatment is still under study. Humans have used cold to treat various conditions for a long time, but whole-body cryotherapy is different because it involves exposure to ultra-cold temperatures that humans don't typically experience. It is also an expensive form of therapy. Is it worth the wellness boost some proponents claim? The jury is still out. If you're considering it, make sure to discuss it first with your healthcare team and proceed with caution. Keep in mind too that you don't have to visit a cryotherapy chamber to get some of the benefits of cold temperatures. A bag of ice remains an effective and inexpensive way to ease the pain of a swollen joint or a sore muscle. And many people swear by a brisk swim in a cold lake or sea as the ultimate energy booster.

Deep breathing

Breathing is one of the most natural and fundamental acts in life. It's a fairly straightforward process: You take in oxygen to fuel your cells, and you release carbon dioxide waste.

Yet we don't always breathe the same way. During moments of stress, our breathing rate and pattern change. A stressed or anxious person takes shallow breaths, using their chest to move air in and out of their lungs. This rapid, shallow breathing can deepen anxiety by making the physical symptoms of stress worse.

Deep, or relaxed, breathing is a technique that helps you breathe more efficiently. It involves deep, even-paced breathing using your diaphragm — the muscle under your rib cage — to expand your lungs. That's why this technique is sometimes called diaphragmatic breathing or paced breathing. The purpose of deep breathing is to slow your breathing, take in more oxygen and reduce the use of shoulder, neck and upper chest muscles while you breathe.

Deep breathing can decrease the effect of stress on your mind and body. It also can slow your heartbeat and lower or stabilize blood pressure. Many relaxation practices use breathing techniques to promote a state of calm.

Such slow, deep breathing techniques are some of the oldest and simplest practices shown to have a variety of therapeutic effects. We can't avoid all the sources of stress in our lives, but we can develop healthier ways of responding to them. Stress relief is often only a breath away.

TWO TYPES OF BREATHING

There are two basic types of breathing: chest breathing and diaphragmatic breathing.

Chest breathing uses secondary muscles in your upper chest. Chest breathing is helpful in situations of great exertion, such as a sprint. During stressful situations, you may inadvertently resort to chest breathing. This can lead to tight shoulder and neck muscles and even headaches. Chronic stress can increase these symptoms. Chest breathing can make you feel short of breath and anxious.

Diaphragmatic breathing, also called belly breathing or abdominal breathing, comes from the body's dominant breathing muscle, the diaphragm. The diaphragm is a dome-like muscle between the chest and the abdomen. When you practice deep breathing, you take a deep breath of air, pause, exhale and then pause before repeating. Your breaths are slow, smooth and deep.

DIAPHRAGMATIC BREATHING TIPS

Diaphragmatic breathing can be practiced in any position, but it is easiest to learn while lying down.

- Lie on your back on a flat surface or in bed, with your knees bent and your head supported.
- Loosen any tight clothing.
- Relax your shoulder and neck muscles. If you wish, close your eyes.

Place one hand on your upper chest and your other hand below your rib cage. This will allow you to feel your diaphragm move as you breathe. **Pursed-lip breathing** will usually help you develop diaphragmatic breathing.

- Breathe in through your nose (as if you are smelling a rose) for about 2 seconds.
- Purse your lips like you're getting ready to whistle or gently blow out candles on a birthday cake.
- Breathe out very slowly through pursed lips to a count of four.
- Repeat four times.
- As you breathe in, your belly should move outward against your hand. The hand on your chest should remain as still as possible.
- As you breathe out slowly through pursed lips, gently tighten your belly muscles. This will push up on your diaphragm to help get your air out.
- Notice how you feel after doing a few pursed-lip breaths.

Now **breathe in and out through the nose**. Find a breathing rate that is comfortable for you.

- For example, you could slowly breathe in for four counts and out for four counts.
- Or, consider adding a short silent phrase to the breathing: "I am" on the inhalation and "relaxed" on the exhalation.

You can practice deep breathing for 5 to 10 minutes a day. This type of daily practice or habit makes it easier to use the breathing technique when stressful situations arise. You can use this breathing anytime, but especially when you are upset or anxious, have difficulty sleeping or are battling pain.

Research on the effects of deep breathing finds it to be beneficial for a variety of conditions, including stress, mood, asthma and pain.

EFFECTS OF DEEP BREATHING
Practicing deep breathing causes several effects in your body:
- Releasing natural feel-good chemicals, such as endorphins.
- Increasing blood flow to your major muscles.
- Making it easier for your heart to do its work.
- Relaxing muscles that have been bracing against pain.
- Helping your body and mind relax and regain strength and energy.
- Helping you relax by reducing stress chemicals in your brain.
- Providing a focus for your mind, which means less opportunity to think about stressful things.

WHAT THE RESEARCH SAYS
Research on the effects of deep breathing finds it to be beneficial for a variety of conditions, including stress, mood, asthma and pain.

Anxiety and stress
Deep breathing can help decrease anxiety. One study found that deep breathing eased tension, anxiety and fatigue in people receiving chemotherapy for cancer. Other studies have found that slow-paced breathing can help reduce symptoms of stress, anxiety, anger, exhaustion and depression, as well as improve quality of life.

Nausea and vomiting
People who are prone to motion sickness have learned to reduce their symptoms of nausea by practicing deep breathing.

Pain
Several studies found that breathing exercises can help people deal with various forms of pain resulting from medical procedures, including after surgery.

Asthma
Research has found moderate evidence that deep breathing improves quality of life in people who have asthma.

Insomnia

One study outlined a potential mechanism of how deep breathing helps with insomnia. The authors hypothesized that slow breathing through the nose has a direct calming effect on the brain , which can help promote sleep.

Blood pressure

In one study of about 50 adults, researchers found that stepwise paced breathing — a breathing exercise in which you gradually reduce the number of breaths you take in a minute — was able to lower blood pressure.

RISK AND SAFETY CONCERNS

Some people get dizzy the first few times they try deep breathing. If you become lightheaded, temporarily discontinue the breathing exercise and try again at another time.

OUR TAKE

As with many other relaxation techniques, deep breathing is easy to do. It can be done just about anywhere, and it's a cost-effective way to reduce stress and anxiety. Just keep reminding yourself that stress relief is only a breath away. And it can be combined with guided imagery (see next section) or meditation (see pages 148-157).

Guided imagery

Imagine for a moment that you're lying on a warm beach somewhere with the sun twinkling on the clear waves as they fall rhythmically on the shore. How does it make you feel? Guided imagery is a technique based on the idea that the mind and the body are connected, and the mind has the power to help regulate physical reactions.

During guided imagery, people imagine being in a pleasant, relaxing space. They build this desirable image in their mind with as much detail as possible, so they can feel, see, hear and smell it as if it were reality.

Scientists have found that imagining in this way typically activates the same parts of the brain that would be involved if it were a real-life occurrence. As these pleasant moments are experienced in the mind, the brain sends messages to the body that influence a wide range of body functions, including heart rate and blood pressure. This practice can ease tension and help a person relax.

Guided imagery is part of mainstream medical practice. It is used by clinicians, psychologists, social workers and other healthcare professionals. You can use the technique by listening to audio versions or following an instructor.

HOW TO PRACTICE GUIDED IMAGERY

Use your imagination to take you to a calm, peaceful place. Try the following steps.

1. Find a comfortable place to sit or lie down. Close your eyes.
2. Take a few deep breaths by breathing in slowly through your nose and letting the air out through your mouth. Let tension flow out of your body with each breath.
3. Picture a calm and peaceful setting. It could be a beach, a garden, a forest, a meadow or any other scene that you like. It could be a favorite spot from your past, a place you went to recently on vacation or someplace you have never been before but would like to visit.
4. Add some detail to your scene. Imagine the sounds, smells, sights and feelings. Is there a breeze? How does it feel on your skin? What do you smell? What does the sky look like? Is it a clear blue sky, or are there clouds? It helps to add a path to your scene. For example, if you're entering a forest, imagine a path leading you through. As you follow the path farther into the woods, continue to release the tension in your body.

5. Take a few minutes to breathe slowly and feel the calm. It's best to do it when you are deep into your scene and are feeling relaxed.
6. Think of a "return" cue, a simple word or sound that you can use in the future to help you return to this place.
7. When you are ready to exit, slowly bring yourself out of the scene and back to the present. Tell yourself that you will feel relaxed and refreshed, and that you'll take the sense of calm you experienced in your imagined place back into reality with you.
8. Count to three and open your eyes. Notice how you feel right now.

Another type of guided imagery is color imagery. It's typically used to release daily hassles and tensions by imagining the tension as a color that changes from red to blue. Think of the color blue as your cue to relax. Follow these steps:

1. Close your eyes and scan your body for tension or discomfort. Picture the color red and associate it with this tension. Imagine all the tense parts of your body as red.
2. Take a deep breath and change the color from red to blue. Imagine the tension melting away as the areas of your body change from red to blue. Feel how the relaxation associated with the color blue settles in.
3. Now imagine the color blue getting deeper and darker. Follow these deepening shades of blue to relax further and further.

WHAT THE RESEARCH SAYS

Evidence suggests that guided imagery may be an effective tool for coping with surgery, cancer treatment, anxiety, pain, insomnia and performance anxiety.

Around surgery

Research indicates that practicing guided imagery before surgery can reduce fear and anxiety. It also can relieve pain following the surgery, leading to earlier discharge times.

In one report, two weeks prior to cardiac surgery patients were given audiotapes to listen to narrated stories set to music. The stories helped guide them to a place in their minds where they felt safe, protected, supported and relaxed. On the day of the surgery, patients brought the audiotapes with them to the hospital and listened to them all the way through to anesthesia. After surgery, their headsets were put back on so that they woke up to the soothing music and continued listening to it afterward. Compared with patients who didn't use guided imagery, their anxiety levels improved by more than 40%. They also needed less medication and went home earlier than those who didn't use guided imagery.

Cancer treatment

In a small study of adults ranging in age from 18 to 72 years who had cancer-related pain, more than half said that guided imagery helped relieve their pain. Those who felt that guided imagery was useful said that the exercise helped distract them from their pain. Some said that the voice leading the exercise was soothing; for others, the imagery involved in the exercise got them to focus on something other than the pain they were feeling. Still others felt that the most useful part of guided imagery was simply the relaxation it brought. Guided imagery has also been used to reduce cancer-related nausea.

Two studies of cancer patients found that guided imagery not only helped ease pain but also reduced their heart rate and blood pressure. Another study found that a combination of guided imagery and Reiki reduced pain and fatigue in cancer patients. Read more about Reiki on page 193.

Anxiety, pain and sleep

A small study recommended guided imagery as a cost-effective method to manage anxiety and pain in people with COVID-19. Another small study found that guided imagery can improve sleep quality in some people.

Enhancing performance

Guided imagery can help with performance. In one study of 62 high school students, participants undertook an eight-week program that taught them cognitive skills they could use to help improve their music performance and reduce their performance anxiety. When they took time to imagine and visualize an upcoming performance, the students felt less anxious about their actual performances.

OUR TAKE

Guided imagery is a useful therapy for treating a variety of health problems. It provides benefits and poses virtually no risk. Guided imagery is used in many medical settings to help manage an array of conditions and diseases from stress to pain to the side effects of cancer. It is also a very cost-effective therapy that can be self-administered in nearly any setting, which makes it a useful tool in any person's wellness toolbox.

Healing touch

Healing touch is an energy-based therapy, like acupuncture (see page 64), that focuses on the flow of "life energy" within the body. Practitioners believe that healing touch can help remove blockages thought to cause discomfort and disease and restore the body's energy balance.

Healing touch practitioners perform an assessment of a person's energy field by moving their hands a few inches above the entire length of the body. This allows practitioners to identify energy blockages and imbalances. Practitioners then use energy techniques to strengthen and manipulate energy fields based on the person's needs.

A MODERN TECHNIQUE

Unlike more ancient methods such as Reiki (see page 193), healing touch is a fairly recent development. Healing touch began in the nursing profession as a contemporary holistic healing practice. It was pioneered in the early 1980s by Janet Mentgen, a nurse who developed her own methods of restoring and balancing energy in her patients.

In 1989, Mentgen formally created healing touch as an energy medicine program and four years later founded the Colorado Center for Healing Touch, dedicated to making the therapy widely available. In 1996 Healing Touch International Inc. (HTI) was formed as an educational and professional membership organization that works to promote the therapy as a holistic form of healing. HTI offers training and certification.

Mastering healing touch techniques involves five levels of training, during which students learn increasingly complex practices and earn a

Many small studies of healing touch have suggested that it's effective for treating certain conditions such as pain, anxiety and fatigue. It also may provide relaxation benefits to those who have undergone certain types of surgery and medical procedures.

diploma if they demonstrate appropriate competency. Students learn how healing touch can be used to calm anxiety, reduce depression and pain, strengthen the immune system, enhance recovery from surgery, ease acute and chronic conditions, aid in neck and spine problems, and support cancer care.

Healing touch also can be used to enhance resilience and a sense of well-being. Students study practical applications such as rebalancing a person's energy fields, clearing blockages and other interventions.

Healing Touch International has over 2,000 members, with more than 200 certified instructors and nearly 2,000 certified HT practitioners. Worldwide, estimates suggest that more than 67,000 individuals, mostly healthcare professionals, have taken healing touch classes.

Interest in healing methods that are rooted in universal energy, sometimes referred to as a person's "biofield," has been growing among patients as well. In a National Health Interview Survey, close to 4 million adults in the United States report having seen a practitioner for energy healing therapy.

HEALING TOUCH AT MAYO CLINIC

Mayo Clinic introduced healing touch into its practice over a decade ago.

Prompted by requests from patients who were interested in more holistic therapies, Mayo Clinic ran its first healing touch and Reiki program, in which several nurses learned healing touch skills. The pilot program lasted six months, during which 133 patients experienced healing touch or Reiki, with several patients receiving multiple treatments, for a total of 144 visits. The primary reasons for treatment were pain, anxiety, nausea and sleeplessness. The pilot went well, so Mayo Clinic nurses began offering this service to patients through a volunteer program. Nurses trained in healing touch provide services and also explain to patients how energy healing works.

"We want to support patient interest for what would help them manage their symptoms or what is important to them," says Susanne M. Cutshall, a clinical nurse specialist at Mayo. Today, patients and their healthcare team can make requests for the service, on an inpatient or outpatient basis.

WHAT TO EXPECT DURING A HEALING TOUCH SESSION

During a session, the healing touch practitioner holds their hands over the recipient's body in specific places that correspond to chakras — the body's spiritual or energy centers. The practitioner typically starts with the feet and moves upward toward the head.

The practitioner may focus on certain places more than others, especially if there are "pain drain" areas that have greater energy needs, explains Susanne M. Cutshall, a clinical nurse specialist at Mayo Clinic. "They may focus on one particular area and do different techniques there," she added. Recipients often describe a deep sense of relaxation during and after a session.

WHAT THE RESEARCH SAYS

Many small studies of healing touch have suggested that it's effective for treating certain conditions such as pain, anxiety and fatigue. It also may provide relaxation benefits to those who have undergone certain types of surgery and medical procedures. One study found that children who are hospitalized on an ongoing basis benefit from receiving healing touch therapy. In another study, researchers found that those who deliver healing touch find benefit in the practice, as well as those who receive the therapy.

Recently, researchers at the cardiac unit of a midwestern acute care hospital piloted a two-month-long healing touch program. During the pilot, the therapy was performed by a certified practitioner and was available to any patient who consented to receive it. The study evaluated the effects of healing touch on pain, nausea and anxiety. It concluded that implementing the program in the acute care setting could bring benefits. More research is needed to identify how to maximize healing touch benefits.

OUR TAKE

The observed benefits of healing touch include relaxation as well as decreased anxiety and pain. However, beyond that, there's limited scientific evidence that healing touch improves health, even though it's used for a variety of medical conditions. Since there's not much risk involved in receiving healing touch therapy, there's little harm in trying it.

Herbs and supplements

Long before modern pharmacological science was developed, people relied on plants and plant extracts to treat a variety of health problems. Some of the earliest mentions of plants being used for medicinal purposes are found in ancient Chinese and Egyptian writings, as far back as 3,000 B.C.E. Indigenous peoples around the globe have a rich history of using herbs and other plants in healing rituals.

Today, the World Health Organization estimates that 80% of people worldwide rely on herbal medicines for some of their healthcare needs. Growth in the herbs and supplements market has led to challenges navigating the safety and efficacy of these substances. This section tells you what is known so far about some common herbs and supplements.

FISH OILS

Fish oils are a dietary source of omega-3 fatty acids, which are necessary for many functions, from muscle activity to cell growth. Your body can't make omega-3 fatty acids, so you have to get them from either food or supplements. Fish oil contains two omega-3s called docosahexaenoic acid (DHA) and eicosapentaenoic acid (EPA). Dietary sources of DHA and EPA are fatty fish, such as salmon, mackerel and trout, and shellfish, such as mussels, oysters and crabs.

"Two to three servings of fatty fish per week seems to serve that general need," says Linda Huang, Pharm.D., R.Ph., a clinical pharmacist at Mayo Clinic. Scientists are also studying whether fish oils can help reduce inflammation and improve memory, she adds. Research has found some evidence that fish oils may lower triglycerides.

GLUCOSAMINE AND CHONDROITIN

Glucosamine and chondroitin are basic building blocks of cartilage, tissue that makes up part of our joints. Some studies found that glucosamine and chondroitin supplements offer benefits for people with osteoarthritis, particularly when it affects the knees. There's also some evidence that they may help with osteoarthritis of the hand and the temporomandibular joint (TMJ) or the jaw. Research is ongoing.

"My typical recommendation [for patients with osteoarthritis] is to try 1,500 milligrams of glucosamine and 1,200 milligrams of chondroitin and then give it 8 to 12 weeks to see whether you find a distinct benefit," says

Dr. Huang. "Many people tell me that they are not sure whether it works, but when they stop it, they feel that their joint aches and pains get worse." Glucosamine rarely causes increases in blood sugar. Glucosamine and chondroitin may interact with other medications, so if you're considering taking these supplements, discuss the decision with your healthcare team.

MELATONIN
Melatonin is a hormone that your brain produces in response to darkness. Taking it can help some people fall asleep. "It does seem that melatonin is able to help with sleep for some individuals," says Dr. Huang, but scientists don't have a full grasp on the optimal dose and the melatonin release process in the body. For example, some melatonin supplements release quickly into the bloodstream. Others are designed to release slowly over time so the effect lasts longer. And there's not enough strong evidence about the effectiveness or safety of melatonin supplements for chronic

EXPERT INSIGHT
HERBS AND SUPPLEMENTS AT MAYO CLINIC

Walk into a store and you'll likely face rows of supplements marketed to cure almost any ailment, from allergies to chronic diseases. While some claims might be valid, many aren't backed by research or haven't been studied enough to make assertions. Often, it's unclear if a particular substance will interact with medications or other substances, such as alcohol. How do you decide what to try?

That's where Linda Huang, Pharm.D., R.Ph., a clinical pharmacist at Mayo Clinic, comes in. Dr. Huang works closely with Brent A. Bauer, M.D., director of research for Mayo's Integrative Medicine and Health program, to help assess the general safety of herbs and supplements and identify interactions between prescription drugs and supplements.

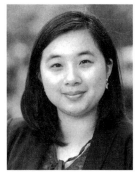

Linda Huang, Pharm.D., R.Ph.
Clinical pharmacist

insomnia. Taking melatonin on a daily basis isn't recommended, especially since there are other ways to improve sleep. (Read about sleep on page 25.)

COENZYME Q10 (COQ10)

Coenzyme Q10 (CoQ10) is an antioxidant that your body produces for cellular growth and maintenance. Lower-than-usual levels of CoQ10 have been found in people with certain conditions, such as heart disease, and in those who take cholesterol-lowering drugs such as statins. Levels of CoQ10 decrease with age. While CoQ10 is found in meat, fish and nuts, this amount isn't enough to significantly increase CoQ10 levels in your body. Studies have found that a CoQ10 supplement can be helpful for heart conditions, diabetes, migraines and the muscular aches and pains caused by statins. Because CoQ10 is involved in energy production, there's a common belief that it might improve physical performance. However, research in this area has produced mixed results.

SAW PALMETTO

Saw palmetto comes from a shrub-like palm native to the southeastern United States. It's commonly marketed for enlarged prostate gland (also called benign prostatic hyperplasia), chronic pelvic pain, migraine, hair loss and other conditions. Several studies — including two large ones funded by the National Institutes of Health — evaluated various preparations of saw palmetto. So far, results are inconclusive. But saw palmetto doesn't appear to cause serious harm either. It generally doesn't interact with other medications or produce concerning side effects, except for mild digestive symptoms or headache in some cases.

GARLIC

Cultivated all over the world, garlic is known for its immune-boosting properties and other health effects. Research suggests that garlic has anti-inflammatory properties and can even pack a cancer-protective punch, especially against colorectal cancer. "High doses of garlic may have a blood-pressure-decreasing effect. It also has a slight blood-thinning effect," says Dr. Huang. "But whether a high dose of garlic is needed and how much it boosts the immune system, I would say it's still in question."

GINKGO

Ginkgo extract, derived from the leaves of the *Ginkgo biloba* tree, is often touted as a memory aid. "Ginkgo has a blood-thinning effect," explains Dr.

Huang, so it could promote circulation in the brain. Yet so far it's not clear whether *Ginkgo biloba* extract can slow or prevent age-related memory problems, or memory loss associated with mild cognitive impairment or Alzheimer's disease.

Several small studies showed modest improvements in cognitive function for older adults with dementia, but larger ones haven't confirmed the findings. One systematic review concluded that it may be helpful for some types of dementia, but overall the jury is still out.

TURMERIC AND CURCUMIN

Turmeric is a common spice often used to add a rich golden color to rice, stews and other foods. It comes from a flowering plant in the ginger family. The active ingredient in turmeric is curcumin, which seems to have anti-inflammatory, antioxidant and even anticancer effects.

Some small studies found it to be effective in providing some improvement in joint pain, reducing anxiety and depression, and decreasing triglycerides and cholesterol. Researchers are delving into the effect of curcumin on cancer because of its anti-inflammatory properties. They also are studying turmeric's effect on diabetes, inflammatory bowel disease and Crohn's disease.

"Turmeric is becoming a very popular topic. It's rising to the top of the list of supplements that people are interested in," says Dr. Huang. "I am seeing it recommended by providers more often for inflammatory disorders, and for pain, especially for patients whose pain who could not be treated with nonsteroidal anti-inflammatory drugs."

GINSENG

Ginseng has long been used in traditional Chinese medicine as a natural energy booster. A Mayo Clinic study found that high doses of a specific type of ginseng, called American ginseng, reduced cancer-related fatigue in people more effectively than a placebo. "Ginseng seems to have stimulant effects, so you have to make sure that you're taking it during the daytime," Dr. Huang says — otherwise you may be too energetic to wind down in the evening.

You also want to watch for which type of ginseng you choose because different properties are associated with different types of ginseng, she adds. This aspect makes it hard to study the herb. Certain types of ginseng might have contaminants that could increase estrogen levels, which isn't good for people with hormonally sensitive breast cancer. If you are considering taking ginseng, talk it over with your healthcare team.

ST. JOHN'S WORT

St. John's wort is a flowering shrub native to Europe. Its flowers and leaves contain a substance called hyperforin, which has been shown to have an antidepressant effect. Several studies found that St. John's wort can help in treating mild to moderate depression. In fact, some research has shown the supplement to be as effective as several prescription antidepressants, so it could be a good option for people who don't want to use pharmaceutical-level antidepressants, Dr. Huang says. However, St. John's wort is not without problems, she adds. It is known to interact with many medications, so it must be taken with caution and only after a conversation with your healthcare team. "It can impact a high number of prescription medications."

FLAXSEED AND FLAXSEED OIL

Flaxseed and flaxseed oil are rich sources of the essential fatty acid alpha-linolenic acid — a heart-healthy omega-3 fatty acid. Flaxseed is high in soluble fiber and in lignans, which contain phytoestrogens, a plant form of estrogen that may have anticancer properties. Flaxseed oil doesn't have phytoestrogens.

There's evidence that flaxseed might reduce cholesterol and may help some people diagnosed with heart and blood vessel diseases. Research also suggests that flaxseed may improve blood sugar levels in some people with type 2 diabetes. It is not known whether flaxseed oil might have such effects. Both flaxseed and flaxseed oil supplements seem to be well tolerated in limited amounts. Few side effects have been reported.

VALERIAN

Results from multiple studies indicate that valerian — a tall flowering grassland plant — may reduce the amount of time it takes to fall asleep and help you sleep better. Of the many valerian species, only the carefully processed roots of *Valeriana officinalis* have been widely studied. Not all studies have shown valerian to be effective, and its use may present risk. For example, an appropriate dose has yet to be identified. In other words, it's unclear how much should be taken and for how long. Although valerian is thought to be fairly safe, side effects such as headache, dizziness, stomach problems and sleeplessness may occur. Additionally, valerian may increase the effects of other sleep aids and the sedative effect of alcohol and certain medications. It also can interfere with some prescription medications and interact with other supplements, such as St. John's wort. If you are on another sedating medication, the addition of valerian might overwhelm your system, Dr. Huang cautions.

GINGER

Ginger has been widely used throughout history both as a spice and as an herbal medicine. It's believed to have many natural medicinal properties and has been used to treat a variety of gastrointestinal symptoms, such as nausea, vomiting, diarrhea and dyspepsia, as well as other ailments, such as arthritis, muscular aches and fever. Today it is more commonly used for nausea and vomiting — two common side effects of chemotherapy treatment. There's evidence that, when taken with standard anti-nausea medications, ginger may help chemo-related gastrointestinal problems.

ZINC

Zinc is a nutrient that aids metabolism and the immune system. Zinc is also important to wound healing and the sense of taste and smell. With a varied diet, your body usually gets enough zinc from chicken, red meat and fortified cereals.

Evidence suggests that if zinc lozenges or syrups are taken within 24 hours after cold symptoms start, the supplement can help shorten the length of colds. Possibly it works by preventing viruses from attaching onto cells, explains Dr. Huang. However, zinc isn't without side effects. It can decrease the effectiveness of certain medications. Also, the use of zinc-containing nasal spray has been linked with a loss of the sense of smell, in some cases long-term or permanently.

IRON

Iron is a mineral the body needs to produce red blood cells. When the body doesn't get enough iron, it can't produce the number of normal red blood cells needed to keep you in good health. This condition is called iron deficiency or iron deficiency anemia. Lack of iron may lead to unusual tiredness, shortness of breath, a decrease in physical performance and learning problems in children and adults. It also may increase your chance of getting an infection.

It's possible to get enough iron from foods such as meat, eggs and leafy green vegetables, but some people need more. Women with heavy periods are at risk of iron deficiency anemia because they lose blood during menstruation. A simple blood test can let you know if you're deficient in iron.

RISKS AND SAFETY CONCERNS

Some herbs and supplements may have side effects that are unpleasant or even harmful. They also may interact with medications you're taking. Herbs and supplements are not reviewed or approved by the U.S. Food

SUPPLEMENTS AND THE FDA

Unlike prescription drugs, herbs and supplements do not require approval from the FDA to be marketed to the public. As such, herbs and supplements don't typically undergo the same type of rigorous clinical trials that prescription drugs do. That's part of the reason there's not always a lot of scientific evidence to show that supplements work.

The FDA does regulate how dietary supplements are manufactured, however, based on the Dietary Supplement Health and Education Act of 1994. The FDA has published specific guidelines for makers of herbs and supplements called Good Manufacturing Practices. These guidelines represent a system for ensuring that products are consistently produced and controlled according to quality standards. For example, the practices outline rules for packaging and labeling dietary supplements, and for avoiding harmful contaminants.

The FDA guidelines also detail what manufacturers can and cannot state on bottles and in advertisements. Unlike prescription drugs, which have specific indications for diseases they're approved to treat, herb and supplement makers cannot state that their products can treat, diagnose, mitigate, prevent or cure disease. However, they can say that their products "may help" with certain conditions, such as pain, or "may promote" certain functions, such as sleep. Because direct causative links haven't been established, manufacturers must use specific language to inform consumers that their product may or may not help with certain ailments.

and Drug Administration (FDA), which presents another problem — as a consumer, you don't necessarily know what's inside the actual pills (see above). "You don't always know whether what's *on* the bottle is a good representation of what we think is *in* the bottle," says Dr. Huang. "It's something we always have to keep in mind."

OUR TAKE
Some herbs and supplements may have beneficial effects for certain conditions. However, most are still being researched, and many studies' results have been inconclusive. If you decide to use herbs or supplements, make sure to discuss it with your healthcare team first to check for potential side effects or interactions with medications.

Homeopathy

In the late 18th century, German physician Samuel Hahnemann came across a bit of information: Supposedly, the quinine-containing bark of the cinchona tree, also called Peruvian bark, cured malaria. Malaria is a potentially fatal infectious disease transmitted by mosquitoes.

Curious, Hahnemann swallowed a dose of Peruvian bark and began to feel feverish, drowsy and thirsty — typical malaria symptoms. As Hahnemann continued to experiment with natural remedies, he developed a theory that "like cures like," meaning that when a substance in large doses causes certain symptoms, in small doses it can cure those same symptoms.

Homeopathy, derived from the Greek words *homeo*, "like," and *patho*, for "disease," is built on this guiding principle. Homeopathic practitioners embrace the idea of treating a person on multiple levels, holding that physical disease also has mental and emotional underpinnings. Therefore, a homeopathic evaluation may take into account physical symptoms, such as fever or pain, along with current emotional and psychological states, such as anxiety and agitation. It may even include an assessment of personality traits, such as creativity, concentration, persistence, sensitivities and other characteristics.

When practitioners devise a remedy, they often take into account all of the above, creating a highly individualized style of medicine. For example, it's common for different people with the same condition to receive different treatments. Three people with migraines can end up with three different remedies.

HOMEOPATHIC PRODUCTS

Homeopathic products come from plants, such as red onion, poison ivy, belladonna, stinging nettle or arnica. They also come from minerals, such as white arsenic. They may come from animals as well, sometimes including even snake venom. Homeopathic products are often made as sugar pellets that are placed under the tongue. But they may come in other forms too, such as ointments, gels, drops, creams and tablets.

Certain methods typically govern the preparation of homeopathic remedies. First, the original ingredients, such as herbs or minerals, are crushed and dissolved in a liquid substance, often alcohol or distilled water. Then these components are mechanically shaken together. The resulting substance is called a mother tincture. Homeopathic

GOOD TO KNOW

Unlike conventional prescription and nonprescription drugs in the United States, which must undergo thorough testing and review by the Food and Drug Administration (FDA) for safety and effectiveness before they can be sold, homeopathic remedies do not have to go through clinical trials.

Products labeled as homeopathic and currently marketed in the United States have not been reviewed by the FDA for safety and effectiveness to diagnose, treat, cure, prevent or mitigate any diseases or conditions. But homeopathic products are regulated by the FDA, which means they must list the active ingredient in the product, the degree of dilution and at least one condition or symptom they are intended to treat.

The guidelines for homeopathic medicines are found in an official guide, the *Homeopathic Pharmacopoeia of the United States,* which is written by a nongovernmental, nonprofit organization of industry representatives and homeopathic experts. The *Pharmacopoeia* also includes provisions for testing new remedies and verifying their clinical effectiveness.

Certain stores and pharmacies sell homeopathic remedies for a variety of problems. Homeopathic practitioners often recommend taking remedies for no more than 2 to 3 days and state that some people may need only 1 or 2 doses before they start feeling better. In some cases, practitioners may recommend daily dosing.

practitioners then dilute tinctures further — once, twice or many times. The process of sequential dilution and shaking is called potentization. Somewhat counterintuitively, homeopathic theory posits that the more diluted the substance, the more potent its healing powers are.

Not surprisingly, homeopathy can be a controversial topic. It's sometimes challenging to reconcile key homeopathic theories with fundamental scientific or medical concepts. For example, in some highly diluted homeopathic preparations the so-called active ingredient can get so scarce that it becomes unmeasurable, which makes the efficacy of the product questionable. It also makes it very difficult to investigate how these products work. Recently, researchers have begun to examine the physical attributes of these preparations to determine if it will be possible to better characterize them.

Despite the challenges, homeopathy is popular. Many people claim to have been helped by homeopathy when conventional medicine didn't work. Based on data from the 2012 National Health Interview Survey, which included a comprehensive survey on Americans' use of holistic therapies, an estimated 5 million adults and 1 million children used homeopathy in the previous year, often for colds and musculoskeletal pain.

FINDING A QUALIFIED HOMEOPATHIC PRACTITIONER
Laws regulating the practice of homeopathy in the United States vary between states. In most states, homeopaths must be licensed healthcare providers. Many homeopathic practitioners are also medical doctors. The American Board of Homeotherapeutics offers such certifications. Naturopathic doctors study homeopathy extensively as part of their medical training, and some are certified by the Homeopathic Academy of Naturopathic Physicians. There are several official homeopathic organizations you can research to find a qualified practitioner:
- The Council for Homeopathic Certification *www.homeopathicdirectory.com*
- The National Center for Homeopathy *www.homeopathycenter.org*
- The American Association of Naturopathic Physicians *www.naturopathic.org*
- The North American Society of Homeopaths *www.homeopathy.org*
- Homeopathic Educational Services in Berkeley, California *www.homeopathic.com*

What happens during a homeopathic consultation
Your first visit to a homeopathic practitioner may take an hour or two, or even longer. Because homeopaths treat the person rather than the illness, they often take their time interviewing new patients, asking many questions and noting personality traits. Some homeopaths also may do a physical examination and possibly order laboratory work.

> Modern medicine doesn't yet understand how homeopathy works, or whether it works. However, a not-so-small number of people believe that it helps their symptoms and improves their health.

THE ORIGINAL NANOMEDICINE?

There are some interesting theories about homeopathy's inner workings. For example, one paper set forth a theory that homeopathy may be the first-ever form of nanomedicine, in which the molecules of active homeopathic ingredients work as tiny nanoparticles that stimulate the body's healing responses. Weaving in molecular physics, the paper's authors argued that as nanoparticles, these molecules have electromagnetic and quantum properties. When they are absorbed by tissues, they can react and interact with other compounds in the body. Ultimately, these nanoparticles can work as "signals" that wake up the body's network of defenses.

That theory has other supporters. Some scientists have posited that the human body functions as a macroscopic quantum system at the molecular level, so the nanoparticles may indeed interact and influence it. Some have proposed updating the term *homeopathy* to *adaptive network nanomedicine*, but that hasn't happened yet.

WHAT THE RESEARCH SAYS

Because homeopathy is so different from other treatments, it is challenging to study from a scientific point of view. Since it aims to treat a specific person, and different people with the same medical problem may get different prescriptions, it can be difficult to design studies and enroll participants.

There is some preliminary evidence for homeopathy's efficacy for certain conditions. For example, individual studies have found that:
- Homeopathic remedies improved subjective measures of menopausal symptoms such as hot flash frequency and severity, mood, fatigue and anxiety.
- Homeopathic dilutions of the plants *Pulsatilla nigricans* and *Thuja occidentalis* worked better than placebo for irritable bowel syndrome.
- Homeopathic treatment for insomnia was more effective than placebo.
- Adding homeopathic medicines to the standard of care for COVID-19 helped people recover more quickly.

However, many other studies have produced inconclusive or unconvincing results on the benefits of homeopathy. Still, this could also mean that modern science has yet to show how homeopathy works.

RISKS AND SAFETY CONCERNS

Generally, homeopathy isn't believed to produce any drastic side effects — in part because many of its remedies are so highly diluted. However, it's possible that some products may contain substantial amounts of active ingredients, which may cause side effects or drug interactions. For example, liquid homeopathic products may contain alcohol, which might be harmful to some. And using homeopathic products containing heavy metals such as mercury also may have harmful effects.

Additionally, some people may experience what practitioners call "homeopathic aggravation" — a temporary worsening of existing symptoms after taking a homeopathic prescription. Researchers have not found much evidence of this reaction in clinical studies; however, research on homeopathic aggravation is scarce.

Certain homeopathic products called "nosodes" or "homeopathic immunizations" have been promoted by some as substitutes for conventional immunizations. But the Centers for Disease Control and Prevention says there's no credible scientific evidence to support such claims. Immunization experts don't recommend replacing vaccinations with homeopathic alternatives.

OUR TAKE

Modern medicine doesn't yet understand how homeopathy works, or whether it works. However, a not-so-small number of people believe that it helps their symptoms and improves their health. Side effects of homeopathy are rare. As long as you're not replacing a proven conventional therapy with homeopathy, it's unlikely to cause significant harm.

If you are interested in using homeopathy for a condition that resists conventional treatments, look for a medical doctor who is also a homeopath. If you are considering using a homeopathic product, bring it with you when you visit your primary healthcare team. They may be able to help you determine if the product poses a risk of side effects or drug interactions for you. And if you develop unusual symptoms while using the product, be sure to discuss these changes with your healthcare team.

Hot tubs and warm pools

Nearly everyone enjoys relaxing in warm water. The warmth of the water eases tight muscles and soothes aches and pains. The water itself lessens the effect of gravity and takes pressure off joints.

Hot tubs are especially made for this form of relaxation, and hot-tubbing is a widely enjoyed form of recreation. Hot tubs are commonly found in hotels, gyms and spas, as well as private homes.

Soaking in a hot tub isn't just a pleasant experience. It also can confer certain tangible health benefits that were not lost on practitioners of ancient medicine. Greek physician Hippocrates, for example, believed that disease resulted from an imbalance of bodily fluids and that bathing, perspiration, walking and massage helped restore biological harmony. In those times, bathing was more than a simple hygienic measure; it was a way to fend off disease. (For more on the history of baths, see page 133.)

Today, health and wellness spas are a $20 billion industry in the United States. There are also medical spas, which are a cross between the traditional day spa and a medical clinic. Medical spas blend the best of two worlds — a relaxing spa experience with the procedures and expertise typically found at a clinic. According to the American Med Spa Association, in 2022 there were 8,841 medical spas in the country.

Recognizing the holistic value of hot tubs and warm pools, Mayo Clinic offers such experiences in its Rejuvenate Spa. Read more about the Rejuvenate Spa and its services here: *healthyliving.mayoclinic.org/rejuvenate-spa.php*.

WHAT THE RESEARCH SAYS
Studies show that warm water can be particularly beneficial in helping manage conditions that involve pain.

Arthritis
Warm water can be helpful in reducing the pain and stiffness of arthritis. Arthritis experts promote the use of warm water pools as a way to reduce the force of gravity that's compressing a joint. Floating in warm water also helps support sore limbs, decrease swelling and inflammation, and increase circulation — all in just 20 minutes. A variety of studies show that people who have arthritis and take part in warm-water exercise programs 2 or 3 times a week often are able to move more easily and experience significantly less pain. These exercise programs also can provide an emotional boost, improve sleep and may be particularly effective for people who are overweight.

Fibromyalgia

Research finds that immersion in hot or warm water can ease fibromyalgia symptoms. In one study, researchers found that warm-water, pool-based exercise, done twice a week for 12 weeks, helped decrease pain in a group of women living with fibromyalgia. In fact, older women and those who had more intense pain showed the most improvement.

Heart health

Heating up in a hot tub makes your heart beat faster, so in some ways it is similar to exercise. When people were not able to exercise due to closures and lockdowns during the COVID-19 pandemic, one paper suggested that regular hot baths might be an effective alternative to physical exercise to improve cardiovascular fitness.

Immersing yourself in a hot tub also can temporarily lower your blood pressure. The warm water widens blood vessels, which in turn brings down your blood pressure. Once you leave the tub, your blood pressure returns to its normal levels. Mayo Clinic research confirmed that soaking in a hot tub increases your heart rate while lowering your blood pressure.

Sleep and mood

A warm bath an hour or so before bedtime can help you relax and get in the right frame of mind for falling asleep. It also can help your body get ready for sleep. Your body temperature changes throughout the day, going down in the evening. So, heating up in a hot bath and then cooling off when you get out helps to create that vital drop in temperature, signaling to your body that it's time to fall asleep. There's also some evidence that hot baths can have antidepressant effects.

RISKS AND SAFETY CONCERNS

Hot tubs aren't for everyone. For people who naturally have low blood pressure, a condition called hypotension, the hot water can lower it too much. Another problematic condition is pulmonary hypertension, which is a type of high blood pressure that affects the arteries in the lungs and the right side of the heart. People with pulmonary hypertension generally should not stay in hot tubs or saunas for too long to avoid having their blood pressure drop too low, which can cause fainting or even death. Hot tubs also aren't recommended if you're pregnant because of the increased risk of certain birth defects.

Another potential, albeit rare, complication of using a hot tub is a condition called "hot tub lung." This condition causes coughing, shortness of breath and fever. It's caused by bacteria inhaled from a hot tub. When not cared for properly, hot tubs can be breeding grounds for dozens of types

> **? DID YOU KNOW?**
>
> Having learned the wisdom of lounging in water pools from the Greeks, the Romans were famous for their baths. Roman baths served as places of recuperation for wounded soldiers but also as rest and recreation centers for the healthy.
>
> Rome boasted three different types of baths: home baths, called *balnea*; private baths, called *balnea privata*; and public baths, called *balnea publica*, which were run by the state. With the introduction of aqueducts, the public baths later developed into huge and impressive bathing centers capable of serving thousands of people. Treatments included applying water to afflicted parts of the body, drinking water and soaking in water, particularly for those with rheumatic and urogenital diseases. Bathing was often combined with sports and education.
>
> With the fall of the Roman Empire, bathing culture fell into disrepute and bathing was officially prohibited. It reemerged during the Renaissance period and eventually spread throughout Europe. In the 1800s, interest in bathing grew along with the belief that bathing in thermal and mineral waters was beneficial for many health ailments. Hotels and guesthouses near hot springs became popular in Europe and North America. Spa resorts became a destination, some even featuring additional attractions such as theaters and casinos.

of bacteria, including potentially harmful ones. For example, one recent study described a case of bacterial pneumonia caused by the inhalation of *Legionella* bacteria, also known as Legionnaires' disease. The bacterial culprit was traced back to a seawater-filled whirlpool in a hotel and spa complex.

Take proper precautions when using a hot tub. Make sure it's been properly sterilized using chlorine. According to the Centers for Disease Control and Prevention, a properly maintained hot tub should give off a faint smell of chlorine. Lastly, the water temperature should not exceed 104 degrees F.

OUR TAKE
As with any therapy, hot tubs and warm pools can have both positive and negative effects. If you're interested in trying a hot tub, talk with your healthcare team first to make sure that it's safe for you. If it is, and if you enjoy it, you may have found another piece of your wellness routine.

Hypnotherapy

Hypnotherapy, also called hypnosis, is a type of therapy designed to lead to a changed state of awareness and increased relaxation, a frame of mind that allows for improved focus and potentially a mental reset. This mental state is often described as one in which a person's typical critical or skeptical nature is bypassed, allowing for acceptance of suggestions.

During hypnosis, the conscious mind may be distracted or guided to become dormant while the subconscious mind enters a suggestible state. As a result, hypnosis typically makes people more open to behavior changes, such as quitting smoking or losing weight. Hypnosis also can help reduce the perception of pain — a concept known as hypnotic analgesia. During hypnosis, most people feel calm and relaxed.

As a practice, hypnosis isn't new. Its origins date back to the ancient Greek temples of Asclepius, where priests spoke to sleeping patients to provide advice and reassurance.

Today, hypnosis is used in a variety of settings, such as hospitals, dental offices and therapy sessions. It's usually done under the guidance of a licensed therapist using verbal repetition and mental images. Although you're more open to suggestions during hypnosis, you don't lose control over your behavior during a hypnosis session. Research finds that the efficacy of hypnosis is very individualized and depends on the specific technique, language and mental imagery hypnotherapists use.

WHY IT'S DONE

One of the main functions of hypnosis today is to help people gain control over behaviors they'd like to change. Hypnosis has been used to help people stop smoking, for example. It's also been used for weight loss. In some cases, it may help you cope better with anxiety or pain. It may ease stress and anxiety before a medical procedure, such as a breast biopsy.

Hypnosis may also be helpful for:

- **Pain control** Hypnosis may help with pain due to burns, cancer, irritable bowel syndrome, fibromyalgia, jaw problems, dental procedures, headaches and childbirth.
- **Hot flashes** Hypnosis may ease hot flashes caused by menopause.
- **Behavior change** Hypnosis has been used with some success to treat sleep problems, bed-wetting, smoking and overeating.
- **Cancer treatment side effects** Hypnosis has been used to ease side effects from chemotherapy and radiation treatment.

- **Mental health conditions** Hypnosis may help reduce anxiety associated with fears and phobias.

WHAT THE RESEARCH SAYS

Several studies have investigated whether hypnosis has a role in contemporary medicine. The findings vary, but it appears that people treated with hypnosis experience substantial benefits for various medical conditions.

Chronic pain

Support for hypnosis as a treatment for chronic pain has boomed recently. Clinical trials found that hypnosis is superior to placebo treatments for chronic pain and has measurable effects on brain areas known to be involved in processing pain.

Hypnotic treatments may have positive effects beyond pain control. For example, hypnotic analgesia in one study had certain measurable effects on brain and spinal cord functioning that differed from the specific hypnotic suggestions therapists made to patients.

Researchers have found the effectiveness of hypnosis to be variable, however. One systematic review examined 85 different trials and found that hypnosis's pain-relieving effects depended on the suggestions and imagery hypnotherapists used — such as suggesting imagining pain as a dial that can be dialed back to reduce or "turn off" pain.

Postoperative pain

Medical hypnosis has been useful in the operating room. One study found that hypnosis might be helpful for postoperative pain — such as after breast cancer surgeries. The results led investigators to suggest it as a potentially useful tool for anesthesiologists. Another study did not find hypnotherapy effective for postoperative pain but found that it helped with fatigue, anxiety and patient satisfaction.

Anxiety

Hypnosis seems to help with some cases of anxiety, but less so in others. One study found hypnosis to be useful for people with chronic obstructive pulmonary disease, who often have difficulty breathing, increased respiratory rate and other anxiety-inducing symptoms. Hypnosis significantly decreased anxiety levels in such people. Another study found that adding hypnosis to standard anxiety therapy offered clear benefits. However, performing a hypnosis session on people undergoing a coronary angiogram — a surgical procedure that uses catheters to get a closer look at blood vessels — did not decrease their anxiety by much.

HOW TO FIND A QUALIFIED THERAPIST
Choose a therapist who is certified to perform hypnosis. If possible, get a recommendation from someone you trust. Learn about any therapist you're considering. Ask questions, such as:
- Do you have specialized training in hypnosis?
- Are you licensed in your specialty in this state?
- How much training have you had in hypnosis? From what schools?
- How long have you done hypnosis?
- What are your fees? Does insurance typically cover your services?

The American Society of Clinical Hypnosis maintains a page where you can search for certified professionals at *www.asch.net/aws/ASCH/pt/sp/find-professional*.

WHAT TO EXPECT DURING A HYPNOSIS SESSION
Wear clothing in which you can settle comfortably and relax. Before you begin, the hypnotherapist will usually explain the process of hypnosis and review your treatment goals. Typically, the therapist begins by talking in a gentle, soothing tone, describing images that create a sense of relaxation, security and well-being.

When you're relaxed and calm, your therapist suggests ways for you to achieve your goals. That may include, for example, ways to ease pain or reduce cravings to smoke. The therapist also may help you visualize vivid, meaningful mental images of yourself accomplishing your goals. At the end of the session, you may be able to bring yourself out of hypnosis on your own. Or your therapist may help you gradually and comfortably increase your alertness.

Contrary to what you might see in movies or during a hypnotist stage act, people don't lose control over their behavior during hypnosis. They usually remain aware during a session and remember what happens.

 Research finds that the efficacy of hypnosis is very individualized and depends on the specific technique, language and mental imagery hypnotherapists use.

Over time, you may be able to practice self-hypnosis. During self-hypnosis, you bring yourself to a state of relaxation without a therapist's guidance. This skill can be helpful in many situations, such as before surgery or other medical procedures. Debbie L. Fuehrer, M.A., L.P.C.C., a mind-body medicine counselor at Mayo Clinic, says that self-hypnosis can be valuable for improving sleep quality, sleep onset and deep sleep. It also can help you go back to sleep after waking in the middle of the night.

RISKS AND SAFETY CONCERNS
Hypnosis done by a trained hypnotherapist is a safe and holistic medical treatment. Be aware, however, that hypnosis may not be safe for some people with severe mental illness. Harmful reactions to hypnosis are rare, but they may include:

EXPERT INSIGHT
HYPNOSIS AT MAYO CLINIC

Mayo Clinic offers hypnosis as a therapy to ease symptoms of many conditions, including stress, anxiety, insomnia and pain. Hypnosis also can lower anxiety before a procedure or surgery.

Debbie L. Fuehrer, M.A., L.P.C.C., is a mind-body medicine counselor at Mayo Clinic. She emphasizes the role of the patient's imagination. "Hypnotic suggestions are present, positive and created with patients using their imagination. The better the patient's use of imagination, the better the hypnosis experience," she says. To ease pain, for example, she suggests that patients release any bodily sensations they do not wish to have while using guided relaxation and replace those unwanted sensations with warmth, strength and calm.

Hypnosis is used at Mayo Clinic as one of the tools in its Integrative Medicine and Health program to help promote physical, mental and spiritual wellness. Specialists integrate hypnosis into an overall treatment plan when it's appropriate.

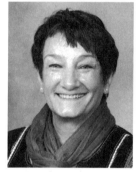

Debbie L. Fuehrer, M.A., L.P.C.C.
Integrative Medicine and Health

- Dizziness
- Headache
- Nausea
- Drowsiness
- Anxiety or distress
- Sleep problems

Additionally, be cautious when someone suggests hypnosis as a way to work through stressful events from earlier in life. That may trigger a strong emotional reaction.

OUR TAKE
When performed by a qualified therapist, hypnosis could be a way to help people cope with pain and reduce stress and anxiety. Hypnosis also may be effective as part of a larger treatment plan for quitting smoking or losing weight. However, hypnosis isn't right for everyone and may not be appropriate for people with severe mental illness. Additionally, not all people are able to enter a state of hypnosis fully enough for it to work well. In general, the more quickly and easily people reach a state of relaxation and calm during a session, the more likely it is that they will benefit from hypnosis.

Massage therapy

One of the oldest wellness practices, massage therapy is a traditional holistic healing method. It is a hands-on technique that involves manipulating soft tissues in the body to reduce stress, ease muscle tension and induce relaxation.

Massage has been used for centuries to heal, soothe and relieve pain. Some sources state that it may go back as far as 5,000 years, taking its origin in the practice of Ayurveda or "science of life" medicine in the Indian subcontinent and spreading from there to China and Egypt. The monks studying Buddhism in China brought massage therapy to Japan, where it became known as shiatsu. The Greeks, who learned the practice from the Egyptians, gave the technique its modern name — the word *massage* comes from the Greek *masso*, which means "to knead."

The Romans also employed massage therapy. Roman physician Galen used massage therapy on emperors, and wealthy Romans enjoyed massages in their homes. Gladiators were given massages to ease pain and muscle fatigue. It is believed that Julius Caesar regularly had his whole body pinched and rubbed down with oils. Homer's *Iliad* and *Odyssey* mention massage with oils and aromatic substances to relax the tired limbs of warriors and help treat wounds.

Today, massage is offered everywhere from luxury spas and upscale health clubs to businesses, hospitals and even airports. *Massage* is a general term for pressing, rubbing and manipulating your skin, muscles, tendons and ligaments. Massage therapists typically use their hands and fingers for massage but also may use their forearms, elbows and even feet. Massage techniques can vary from light stroking to applying deep pressure.

BENEFITS OF MASSAGE THERAPY

Massage is increasingly offered alongside conventional treatment for a wide range of medical conditions and situations. Massage generally makes people feel good, which promotes relaxation and lowers stress.

Physical benefits of massage include:

- Improved circulation
- Decreased muscle stiffness
- Decreased joint inflammation
- Better quality of sleep
- Quicker recovery between workouts

- Improved flexibility
- Less pain and soreness
- Strengthened immune response

Mental benefits of massage include:
- Lower stress levels
- Improved relaxation
- Improved mood
- Decreased anxiety
- More energy
- Increased feeling of wellness

TYPES OF MASSAGE THERAPY

There are approximately 80 massage therapy styles available with a wide variety of pressures, movements and techniques. Here are a few of the most common types of massage.

Swedish massage is a popular technique. It's a gentle form of massage that uses long strokes, kneading, deep circular movements, vibration and tapping to help you feel relaxed and energized.

Deep tissue massage is a technique that uses slower, more forceful strokes to target the deeper layers of muscle and connective tissue. It's commonly used to help with tension and muscle damage from injuries such as back sprains.

Sports massage is geared toward preventing or treating injuries for people involved in sports activities and to promote flexibility.

Shiatsu massage applies pressure on certain points of the body. Called acupressure points, they are important for the flow of qi (CHEE), the body's vital energy, according to traditional Chinese medicine practice. Applying pressure to these points helps remove blockage and restore qi flow.

Thai massage involves compression of muscles, mobilization of joints and acupressure.

In *hot stone massage*, the therapist places warmed stones on certain areas of the body, such as acupressure points. The stones may be used as massage tools or temporarily left in place to transmit heat deep into the body and promote relaxation.

Some of the benefits of massage therapy include improved circulation, decreased muscle stiffness, better sleep, less pain and more energy.

A *lymphatic drainage massage* is a gentle, long-stroke massage of your tissues meant to increase the circulation of lymph fluids, which filter out bacteria, viruses and waste from your body.

Reflexology massage relies on hand, thumb and finger techniques to stimulate certain points on your feet, which are believed to correspond to various parts of the body. It aims to enhance overall health and well-being. For more on reflexology, see page 190.

Cranial massage aims to alleviate headaches, migraines, neck and back pain, temporomandibular joint (TMJ) dysfunction and certain neurological conditions.

Trigger point massage involves applies pressure directly to specific trigger points to release tension and ease pain. The pressure varies in intensity, and the therapist may use their fingers, knuckles and elbows to relax the contracted muscle fibers and increase blood flow, which promotes muscle relaxation.

WHAT TO EXPECT DURING A MASSAGE
No matter what kind of massage you choose, you should feel calm and relaxed during and after your session. When you have a massage, here's what to expect:
- You'll likely need to answer questions about your goals for your massage. For example, are you looking solely to relax or for relief in a specific area? Your massage therapist will also want to know about any medical conditions you might have.
- You may need to undress or wear loose-fitting clothing. Undress only to the point that you're comfortable. You generally lie on a table and cover yourself with a sheet.
- Most of the time, you will lie on your stomach at the beginning of your massage and then transition to a faceup position. If you're unable to lie facedown, your therapist may have you lie on your side. The therapist may use pillows or bolsters to take strain off your lower back and allow you to relax during the massage. You also can have a

massage while sitting in a chair that's specially made to slope forward so that the therapist can work on your back while you're fully clothed.
- Depending on preference, your massage therapist may use oil or lotion to reduce friction on your skin. Tell the therapist if you are allergic to any ingredients or are sensitive to certain scents.

WHAT THE RESEARCH SAYS

Researchers have found that massage is an effective way to reduce stress, pain and muscle tension. It releases endorphins — the body's natural painkillers — and increases blood flow. It also can reduce blood pressure and promote better sleep. More research on the benefits of massage is

EXPERT INSIGHT
MASSAGE FOR PAIN RELIEF

Jennifer L. Hauschulz, a board-certified massage therapist at Mayo Clinic, has seen many patients benefit from her sessions over the past 20 years. Yet there's one case that she remembers specifically.

A 45-year-old woman developed a debilitating pain in her neck and shoulders right after an abdominal hernia surgery. She also complained of having double vision, numbness on the left side of her face and weakness on the left side of her body. Muscular pain and nerve irritation sometimes develop due to a patient's prolonged position during surgery, which may leave them sore, but usually these symptoms resolve themselves. However, the woman's symptoms were so severe that her hospital stay needed to be prolonged.

"On day six, her doctors ordered a massage," Hauschulz recalls. "I started working on her, and her neck began adjusting, and by the end of the massage, her normal vision returned and her tingling sensations went away. All of her symptoms were almost completely gone after one half-hour massage in the hospital. She was able to go home the next day."

While many people may think of massage as a way to pamper themselves, in the hands of a qualified practitioner it can be a potent therapeutic tool. As a massage therapist who works in outpatient settings as well as with people who are hospitalized, Hauschulz has seen the field of massage therapy change and evolve, creating alternatives to needed, but the studies that have been done so far indicate that massage may be helpful in a number of situations.

Pain and anxiety relief
Massage therapy can be effective in the management of acute and chronic pain, and it can serve as a nonaddictive alternative to opioids.

Researchers have found that massage is useful for chronic low back pain and neck pain, rheumatoid arthritis, and various forms of cancer pain. A study looking at treatment options for people with multiple sclerosis found that massage improved sleep and decreased pain, fatigue, and anxiety in this group.

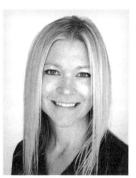

Jennifer L. Hauschulz
Integrative Medicine and Health

painkillers and other medications. "Because of the opioid crisis doctors don't prescribe opioids as much as they used to," Hauschulz says. "Instead, they're prescribing alternatives like massage, acupuncture or physical therapy. And people don't want to take pills for everything either; they are trying to get off medications because medications may have side effects."

Today, both doctors and patients are looking for more holistic healing — and massage can be a safe and effective treatment. Massage is well known for its benefits in relieving pain and stress. But it's also used for a number of other conditions, including digestive disorders, headache and fibromyalgia, as well as after surgery and even alongside cancer treatment.

Many studies have shown that massage offers a range of benefits to people undergoing and recovering from cancer treatment. "In fact, oncology patients can really benefit from massage," Hauschulz says. "When their bodies are undergoing chemo or radiation, they're fatigued, they have brain fog, they may have compromised lymphatic flow and they can develop nerve pain. Massage can help with all of those things."

Researchers at Mayo Clinic also studied the effects of massage on patients who underwent colorectal surgery. They found that postoperative massage significantly improved patients' perception of pain, tension and anxiety. In another Mayo Clinic study, women who underwent mastectomy reported similar massage effects.

Fibromyalgia is a complex condition, characterized by chronic widespread pain often accompanied by anxiety, depression, stiffness and trouble sleeping. A systematic review of medical literature found that fibromyalgia patients who received regular massage therapy for five weeks or longer suffered less from pain, anxiety and depression. The paper recommended massage as a viable fibromyalgia treatment.

Heart health

Mayo Clinic has conducted several studies to discover the most effective uses of massage therapy. In one study, massage therapy was offered to people undergoing heart surgery. This type of surgery often involves a high level of pain because of the location of the incisions, as well as the presence of nerve fibers along the ribs. Breathing causes constant movement in these areas, which adds to the pain — and, in turn, adds to feelings of stress. Massage recipients reported having dramatically lower levels of pain and anxiety. After reviewing the study's conclusions, surgeons made massage therapy a routine part of care following open-heart surgery.

In another study, Mayo Clinic researchers found that a 20-minute massage done 30 minutes before a cardiac catheterization procedure made patients feel less anxious and tense, and reduced pain too.

In addition to helping relieve pain following heart surgery, massage may be therapeutic from a prevention standpoint. Massage therapy has been shown to help with blood pressure and stress management, which can help promote heart health.

Mental health and wellness

Massage therapy offers benefits for a number of mental health conditions, including depression, anxiety and stress. Research also shows that massage can help people cope with seasonal affective disorder by improving mood and boosting energy levels.

Aging

Massage therapy treats the aches and pains of aging and helps manage chronic pain. Researchers have found that regular massage promotes relaxation and stability and even lessens the effects of dementia, high blood pressure and osteoarthritis.

MASSAGE AT MAYO CLINIC

Mayo Clinic has offered massage to patients for nearly two decades as part of its holistic approach to health and healing. But for many years prior, a massage at bedtime was considered routine for hospital patients.

Trained board-certified specialists at Mayo Clinic offer massage therapy for various conditions. Massage therapy techniques can decrease swelling and impaired joint mobility, ease muscle spasms and muscle tension, and increase circulation to promote healing. Massage also can reduce pain and improve muscle tone. The majority of massage offered at Mayo Clinic is Swedish massage, but therapists also perform acupressure, reflexology, mobilization of scar tissue, oncology massage and lymphatic massage.

People staying in the hospital may have wounds from surgery, for example, or they may be connected to medical equipment such as intravenous lines or chest drains. To promote patient wellness and healing, Mayo Clinic has a training program to help massage therapists work with people who are in a hospital.

"We do various types of massage, from very acute care for postsurgery patients to those in chronic pain," says Hauschulz. "We modify our massage techniques and pressure to patients' needs. I also do a lot of scar tissue massage, which is helpful for patients struggling with pain or adhesions from previous surgeries."

Healthcare teams at Mayo Clinic work together to coordinate a massage therapy treatment plan for an injury or condition as part of a person's overall plan of care. Massage therapy may be recommended for conditions such as:

- Postoperative care
- Headache
- Sports injuries
- Soft tissue strains and injuries
- Scar tissue
- Insomnia
- Anxiety
- Depression
- Digestive disorders
- Fibromyalgia
- Nerve pain
- TMJ disorders

Cancer care
Massage may reduce pain, improve mood, promote relaxation and improve sleep in people with cancer. A massage therapist typically takes certain precautions when treating someone with cancer, such as avoiding massaging skin that's being treated with radiation therapy or not massaging directly over a tumor, so finding a skilled therapist is important.

Workplace stress management
The benefits of massage therapy at Mayo Clinic aren't limited to patients. Working in a hospital can be a source of stress, so Mayo Clinic launched a pilot program, offering chair massage for nurses working in stressful environments. For this trial, nurses were given a 15-minute chair massage. Investigators noted a dramatic decrease in stress-related symptoms and anxiety, and almost 80% of the nurses said they felt that their overall job satisfaction improved because of massages.

FINDING A MASSAGE THERAPIST
Several types of healthcare professionals — such as physical therapists, occupational therapists and massage therapists — perform massage. Ask your healthcare team or friends and family for a recommendation. Check online directories that include reviews.

Once you've identified a few professionals who might be a good fit for you, research their credentials. Although not all massage therapists are required to be board certified, you can find a list of board-certified massage therapists in your area by visiting the National Certification Board for Therapeutic Massage & Bodywork's website at *www.ncbtmb.org*. Then find out what they charge and whether your health insurance will cover it.

If you're interested in finding a massage therapist who has experience in working with people who have cancer, the Society for Oncology Massage (*http://s4om.org*) is a helpful resource.

Don't be afraid to ask a potential massage therapist questions such as:
- Are you licensed, certified or registered?
- What is your training and experience?
- How many massage therapy sessions do you think I'll need?
- What's the cost, and is it typically covered by health insurance?

RISKS AND SAFETY CONCERNS
If you have had a recent heart attack, have a bleeding disorder or are taking blood-thinning medication, talk to your doctor or someone on your healthcare team before scheduling a massage. Also check with a medical professional before trying massage if you've had a recent blood clot in

your leg or if you have newer burns, fractures, or severe osteoporosis; massage may be harmful in these cases.

Massage generally isn't performed directly on tumors, and people with healing wounds or nerve damage should avoid pressure on affected areas of the body. Keep in mind that you shouldn't feel significant pain during a massage, although some forms can leave you feeling a bit sore the next day. If a massage therapist is pushing too hard, ask for lighter pressure.

OUR TAKE

Massage therapy is safe and effective for people of all ages. It's not only a feel-good way to pamper yourself. It's also a powerful tool to help you take charge of your health and well-being, whether you have a specific health condition or are looking for a stress reliever.

Almost everyone feels better after a massage. Massage has been shown to help treat many conditions and boost overall wellness in a number of ways. There are different types of massage. If you find one that works for you, you may be surprised at how quickly it can become a regular part of your wellness routine. While generally safe, there are some instances in which massage may not be recommended (see "Risks of massage" on the opposite page).

Meditation and mindfulness

Meditation is one of the oldest known mind-body practices. Rooted in ancient Eastern traditions such as Ayurveda, Taoism and Buddhism, it originally was meant to help deepen understanding of the sacred aspects of life and bring balance to inner consciousness.

It can still do so today. It also can help people increase their well-being and manage chronic illnesses. In modern use, the term *meditation* describes a group of diverse techniques that focus on developing and fine-tuning the mind-body connection.

There are many ways of practicing meditation. Some types of meditation involve maintaining mental focus on a particular sensation, such as breathing, a sound, a visual image or a mantra — a repeated word or phrase. Other forms of meditation include the practice of mindfulness, which involves maintaining attention or awareness of the present moment without making judgments. Prayer can be a form of meditation too. There is also meditation with movement.

In general, the idea behind meditation is to suspend the stream of thoughts that normally occupies your conscious mind. Doing this can lead to a state of physical relaxation, mental calmness and psychological balance.

Programs that teach meditation or mindfulness may add on other practices such as tai chi or yoga (see pages 209 and 218). For example, mindfulness-based stress reduction is a program that teaches mindful meditation, but it also includes discussion sessions and other strategies to help people apply what they have learned to stressful experiences.

Practicing meditation can change how you relate to the flow of your emotions and thoughts, and it may help you control how you respond to a challenging situation. For example, if you're claustrophobic and you know you're going to have an MRI, meditating and focusing on your breathing as you inhale and exhale may help you feel less anxious and get through the exam. Or maybe public speaking makes you feel nervous. Taking five deep breaths before giving an important presentation may help you slow down, relax and focus.

Anyone can practice meditation. It's simple, free and doesn't require any special equipment. In addition, meditation is a type of holistic medicine that you can practice wherever you are — whether you're out for a walk, riding the bus, waiting at the doctor's office or even in the middle of a tense business meeting.

148   Mayo Clinic Guide to Holistic Health

HOW TO PRACTICE MEDITATION AND MINDFULNESS

There is no right or wrong way to practice meditation and mindfulness. You can make it as formal or informal as you like, however it suits your lifestyle and situation. Some people build meditation into their daily routine — for example, starting and ending each day with time for meditation. Others try to incorporate mindfulness throughout the day, regularly pausing to bring their attention back to the sights, sounds and smells around them.

Other options for centering your awareness include listening to sacred music, spoken words or any music you find relaxing or inspiring. You may want to write your reflections in a journal or discuss them with a friend or spiritual leader.

Meditation

Here are some common techniques for engaging in meditation.

Body scan meditation Lie on your back with your legs extended and arms at your sides, palms facing up. Focus your attention slowly and deliberately on each part of your body, in order, from head to toe. Be aware of sensations, emotions or thoughts associated with each part. "The body scan is a very simple way of being present with your body and whatever is happening right now," says Roberto P. Benzo, M.D., a pulmonologist and founding director of the Mindful Breathing Laboratory at Mayo Clinic.

Sitting meditation Sit comfortably with your back straight, feet flat on the floor and hands in your lap. Breathing through your nose, focus on your breath moving in and out of your body. If physical sensations or thoughts interrupt your meditation, note the experience and then return your focus to your breath. For many of us, sitting down and being quiet can be really hard, Dr. Benzo says, but when you try sitting meditation, it can become quite simple.

Walking meditation Find a quiet place 10 to 20 feet in length and begin to walk slowly. Focus on the experience of walking, being aware of the sensations of standing and the subtle movements that keep your balance. When you reach the end of your path, turn and continue walking, maintaining awareness of your sensations. "This type of meditation is good for restless people who cannot sit still," Dr. Benzo says. "For some people, like me, it's one of the most important practices."

Guided meditation Sometimes called guided imagery or visualization, this method of meditation involves forming mental images of places or situations you find relaxing. You try to imagine using as many senses as possible, such as smells, sights, sounds and textures. You may be led through this process by a guide or teacher.

Love and kindness meditation This form of meditation enables you to connect to the sense of love and kindness that's within you. As you meditate, you grow and develop these feelings inside you, so you become a repository of that love and kindness. "It's really useful to be kind to yourself, especially in the moment of suffering," says Dr. Benzo. "And once you have enough of this kindness, you can give it to others."

Mantra meditation In this type of meditation, you silently repeat a calming word, thought or phrase to prevent distracting thoughts. These can be words that are particularly important to you or just the "om" chant that's used in yoga, says Dr. Benzo. That particular chant can create certain vibrations in the body that align your mind with your body.

Although you don't need equipment to meditate, it helps to get yourself physically and mentally settled before you begin a session.

- **Find a quiet setting** If you're a beginner, practicing meditation may be easier if you're in a quiet spot with few distractions, including no digital devices or television. As you get more skilled at meditation, you may be able to do it anywhere, especially in high-stress situations where you benefit the most from meditation, such as a traffic jam, a stressful work meeting or a long line at the grocery store.
- **Settle into a comfortable position** You can practice meditation whether you're sitting, lying down, walking or doing other activities. Just try to be comfortable so that you can get the most out of your meditation. Aim to keep a posture that brings attention to the present moment.
- **Focus your attention** Focusing your attention is generally one of the most important elements of meditation. Focusing your attention is what helps free your mind from the many distractions that cause stress and worry. You can focus your attention on such things as a specific object, an image, a mantra or just your breathing.
- **Practice conscious breathing** This technique involves deep, even-paced breathing using the diaphragm muscle to expand your lungs. The purpose is to slow your breathing, take in more oxygen and reduce the use of shoulder, neck and upper chest muscles while breathing so that you breathe more efficiently.
- **Keep an open attitude** Let thoughts pass through your mind without judgment.

DID YOU KNOW?

The earliest records of meditation are found in the Vedic religion of the Indo-European people who settled in India around 1500 B.C.E. These people developed the ancient Indian medical system known as Ayurveda, which embraces a natural and holistic approach to physical and mental health. Ayurveda (the term translates as "science of life") relies on medicines from plants and minerals, as well as diet, exercise and lifestyle. One of Ayurveda's principles is that diseases develop due to an imbalance in elements of a person's consciousness. Meditation is an Ayurvedic approach to maintaining that balance. Many other meditative techniques similarly began in Eastern traditions.

In the West today, the word *meditation* has become part of everyday vocabulary. You may hear celebrities talking about meditating and sports figures saying they meditate as part of their exercise routine. There are multiple meditation apps available for smartphones and other digital devices.

The practice continues to increase in popularity. According to a recent survey, the percentage of U.S. adults who practiced some form of meditation — such as mindfulness, mantra-based or spiritual meditation — tripled over a period of five years. At the same time, mindfulness programs for schools have become popular, leading to an increase in the practice among children age 4 to 17. These school programs teach mindfulness to help students and teachers manage stress and anxiety, resolve conflicts, and control impulses as well as improve resilience, memory and concentration.

Mindfulness

Mindfulness involves bringing your attention to the present moment without making any judgement. Doing so may provide you with clarity and compassion for yourself and others. Here are some simple ways to practice mindfulness:

- **Pay attention** In a busy world, it's hard to slow down and notice things. Take the time to experience your environment with all of your senses — touch, sound, sight, smell and taste. For example, when you eat a favorite food, take the time to truly savor it.
- **Live in the moment** Try to bring an open, accepting and discerning attention to everything you do. Find joy in simple pleasures.

MEDITATION AND MINDFULNESS | Therapies A–Z   **151**

- **Accept yourself** Treat yourself the way you would treat a good friend.
- **Focus on your breathing** When you have negative thoughts, try to sit back, take a deep breath and close your eyes. Focus on your breath as it moves in and out of your body. Sitting and breathing for even just a minute can help you return to a nonjudgmental position.

WHAT THE RESEARCH SAYS

Although a growing body of scientific research supports the health benefits of meditation, some researchers believe it's not yet possible to draw conclusions regarding this type of integrative therapy. While many studies have been small and not conducted with the highest degree of rigor, the overall evidence to date supports the use of meditation for a variety of medical conditions.

EXPERT INSIGHT
THE COURAGE OF BEING PRESENT

"Our modern life is very busy," says Roberto P. Benzo, M.D., a pulmonologist at Mayo Clinic. "We are constantly on the go. We have myriad responsibilities, appointments, deadlines and obligations. To top it, everything competes for our attention. We are so bombarded by so many things. We are either on our phones or on our tablets or computers, sending texts, reading emails or checking Facebook. The entire electronics industry is trying to hijack our attention. People's attention is a currency today."

As a result, our minds are preoccupied with all sorts of things and we pay only partial attention to what is going on in the present. "Our mind is constantly somewhere else," Dr. Benzo adds. That makes it hard to focus, stay in the present moment, decompress or release stress. Meditation and mindfulness can help restore a balance between the body and mind, making room for gut and heart feelings to help us make decisions and lead our lives. But while these two concepts go hand in hand, they are not the same thing, Dr. Benzo explains. "Mindfulness is about the awareness we have about what is happening right now, without passing judgments, such as liking or disliking. And meditation is about observing what is actually happening," he says. "There's a close

Emotional and physical well-being

Research suggests emotional and physical benefits of meditation include:
- Gaining a new perspective on stressful situations.
- Building skills to manage stressors in your life.
- Increasing self-awareness.
- Focusing on the present.
- Reducing negative emotions.
- Increasing imagination and creativity.
- Increasing patience and tolerance.
- Lowering resting heart rate.
- Lowering resting blood pressure.
- Improving sleep quality.

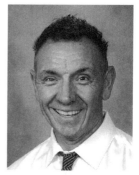

Roberto P. Benzo, M.D.
Pulmonary and Critical Care Medicine

connection between them," he adds, but there are also differences. For example, mindfulness isn't just about meditating. It can be embraced as a way of living too. And while it may not be obvious, mindfulness takes some mettle.

"There is a kind of courage to mindfulness," says Dr. Benzo. That's because so many people often live what he describes as a substitute life. "We want to show that we are perfect and without mistakes and making the right decisions," he says, likening that life to wearing a mask. "We don't show others the real version of ourselves. The thing is that in order to be yourself and be honest and sincere, you have to be courageous." It takes some courage to accept what's happening, he clarifies: "The courage of being present or having a nonjudgmental presence to accept what you cannot change."

Plus, in our busy society it's not very popular to just sit there doing nothing. "Just sitting or just walking or just breathing is not popular," Dr. Benzo says. "But the payback can be huge. The payback is balance."

Disease management

Meditation might also be useful for managing symptoms if you have a medical condition, especially one that may be worsened by stress.

Asthma When practicing mindfulness-based stress reduction for 12 months, adults with mild, moderate or severe persistent asthma experienced significant and lasting improvements in quality of life and stress management even though their lung function didn't necessarily get better.

Heart health and blood pressure A research review found that certain meditative techniques can effectively lower blood pressure in adults and adolescents, and in some cases reduce the need for blood pressure medication. Meditative practice improved cardiovascular function and decreased heart and respiratory rates as well as levels of the stress hormone cortisol.

The authors observed that these easy-to-learn practices were also cost-effective ways for people to improve their health. Overall, meditation was found to have positive effects on the cardiovascular system because it helps reduce stress, a risk factor for heart disease.

Cancer Multiple studies have found that women with breast cancer, as well as people with other cancer types, who practice meditation, mindfulness, yoga or other similar techniques are better able to cope with cancer-related stress, anxiety, depression, fatigue and general distress. Additionally, meditation exercises often improve overall quality of life.

One study found that a meditation-based program was effective in decreasing mood disturbance and stress symptoms for up to six months in people with a wide variety of cancer diagnoses and stages of illness. In another study of people with cancer, the use of relaxation, meditation and yoga improved sleep and quality of life, and reduced stress. Finally, a meta-review of 16 studies involving over 2,000 patients with cancer found that mindfulness practices substantially improved loneliness and depression.

Sleep problems Evidence suggests that meditation practice can improve sleep quality in people experiencing difficulty sleeping. In addition, benefits appear to persist over the long term. Some of the ways meditation might help include calming the mind and reducing thinking processes that interfere with sleep, and having a positive effect on the flow of sleep cycles. Regular practice of meditation may even alter different parts of the brain related to sleep as well as the connections between these part.

MEDITATION AT MAYO CLINIC

Mayo Clinic hosts weekly meditation sessions that are free and open to everyone. "Anyone can join from anywhere," says Dr. Benzo. "It's completely free and we do it every Wednesday."

You can join in on Wednesdays at 5:30 p.m. Central time by visiting *www.mayo.edu/research/labs/mindful-breathing*, and clicking on the "Join a Meeting" link inside the "Live Virtual Meditation" box. If the Wednesday schedule doesn't work for you, you can listen to prerecorded guided meditations when you have a few spare minutes during the day by visiting the website listed above and clicking on "Audio Files."

Mayo Clinic also maintains meditation and spiritual spaces at various locations on its three campuses, which are open to all patients and visitors.

Mayo Clinic in Arizona
- Healing Garden
- Mayo Clinic Hospital Chapel

Mayo Clinic in Florida
- Cahill Meditation Atrium
- Louchery Island

Mayo Clinic in Minnesota
- Chapels and reflective spaces
- Mayo Clinic Hospital, Methodist Campus Chapel
- Mayo Clinic Hospital, Saint Marys Campus Chapel
- Saint Francis Chapel
- Groves Foundation Meditation Room
- Saint Francis Peace Garden
- Mayo Center for the Spirit
- Mayo Building, Subway Level

Anxiety, depression and stress Various mind-body techniques helped frontline workers cope with the challenges of the COVID-19 pandemic. A review of 33 studies found that in 29 of them mindfulness-based practices benefited healthcare workers by increasing well-being, engagement and resilience and reducing burnout. Another review investigated the effects of mindfulness-based interventions on more than 1,300 frontline healthcare workers and found them to be relatively effective in reducing symptoms of anxiety, depression and stress. Overall, meditation seems to reduce various aspects of psychological stress.

Irritable bowel syndrome (IBS) Conventional treatment for IBS is usually aimed at trying to manage symptoms, often through dietary modifications. It isn't always satisfactory. A review of studies investigating mindfulness as a way to help manage IBS found that those who practiced mindfulness experienced less-severe symptoms, less pain and a higher quality of life. Higher quality of life persisted even after the studies ended.

Immune function Although directly linking the effects of meditation to immune function is challenging, some studies suggest that meditation practice can have protective effects. A large-scale genomic study found that people who took part in a meditation retreat had a dramatic change in immune function. They experienced increased activity in over 60 genes related to a molecule called interferon, which helps cells fight off viruses.

During the pandemic, researchers gathered blood samples from experienced meditators after an intensive weeklong meditation exercise. The researchers then measured levels of antiviral proteins in the meditators' blood plasma. The results indicated that meditation enhances resiliency to viral infections and could be a possible aid in the management of COVID-19 in addition to vaccines and other medical treatments.

Similarly, another study concluded that certain types of meditations, such as yoga, could be effective add-on measures for preventing and treating COVID-19 infections.

Meditation and mindfulness can help reduce stress and lower risks for various stress-related disorders. As the evidence supporting the use of meditation grows, adding it to your daily schedule may be just the antidote you need to deal with a hectic routine.

RISKS AND SAFETY CONCERNS

Meditation and mindfulness practices are usually considered to have few risks, but some people do have negative experiences with these practices. In an analysis of studies on more than 6,000 people, about 8% of participants reported negative effects — most commonly anxiety or depression — which is similar to the percentage reported for most psychological therapies.

OUR TAKE

Meditation and mindfulness practices offer a variety of health benefits and may help people not only improve the quality of their lives but also boost their health and immunity. Meditation and mindfulness can help reduce stress and lower risks for various stress-related disorders. The long-term benefits of meditation continue to undergo study.

Multivitamins

The word *vitamin* comes from the Latin word *vita*, which means "life." And vitamins are indeed vital to our health and well-being. Vitamins were first identified in 1912 by Casimir Funk, a Polish chemist who later immigrated to the United States. Before his discovery, scientists believed that only four nutritional factors were essential for good health: proteins, carbohydrates, fats and minerals. At the time, many medical experts also embraced the germ theory of disease and believed that all illnesses were caused by microbes. But some diseases, such as scurvy and pellagra, did not fit this model. While studying these illnesses, Funk isolated forms of vitamin B. His discovery cured pellagra — now known to be a deficiency of niacin, a kind of vitamin B. Following Funk's findings, scientists uncovered many more vitamins, which are now understood to be crucial for good health.

Vitamin and multivitamins are some of the most common supplements available today. Yet, the best way to get your daily dose of vitamins and minerals is still by eating a balanced diet. Because your body needs fairly small amounts of vitamins, you can usually get enough of them through the foods you eat.

But if you need to limit your diet because of food allergies or food intolerances, taking vitamin supplements can make up for dietary deficiencies. Multivitamins are also recommended for vegetarians and vegans who eat no animal products, and for people who are at risk of inadequate nutrition, such as older adults and people who smoke or consume excessive amounts of alcohol.

The next sections explore the most important vitamins your body needs. It is helpful to understand symptoms of a potential vitamin deficiency, how the vitamins interact with body processes, where they can be found in a regular diet and when supplements might be necessary.

VITAMIN B-1

Vitamin B-1 (thiamine) is one of the eight B-complex vitamins that help your body convert food to energy. Lack of thiamine may lead to a condition called beriberi. Signs of beriberi include loss of appetite, constipation, muscle weakness, pain or tingling in arms or legs, and possible swelling of feet or lower legs.

Severe lack of thiamine may cause depression, memory problems, weakness, shortness of breath and fast heartbeat. Your healthcare professional may treat this by prescribing a thiamine supplement for you. You also can find thiamine in various foods, including whole-grain and enriched cereals, peas, beans, nuts, and meats, especially pork and beef. Some dietary thiamine is lost during cooking.

VITAMIN B-3
Vitamin B-3, commonly known as niacin, helps improve blood circulation and cholesterol levels. In high doses, niacin can reduce low-density lipoprotein (LDL, or "bad") cholesterol and triglycerides and raise high-density lipoprotein (HDL, or "good") cholesterol. Despite niacin's ability to raise HDL, research suggests that niacin therapy isn't linked to lower rates of death, heart attack or stroke. High doses of niacin — between 2,000 and 6,000 milligrams per day — can cause liver damage, severe low blood pressure and other serious side effects.

Therefore, high-dose intakes should be considered a prescribed medication, not a vitamin supplement, and taken under medical supervision. The recommended daily amount of niacin for adult males is 16 milligrams a day, and for adult women who aren't pregnant the recommendation is 14 milligrams a day.

VITAMIN B-6
Vitamin B-6 (pyridoxine) is important for normal brain development and for keeping your nervous and immune systems healthy. A healthy and varied diet will provide most people with enough vitamin B-6. Food sources of vitamin B-6 include poultry, fish, potatoes, chickpeas, bananas and fortified cereals.

People who have kidney disease or conditions that interfere with absorbing nutrients from foods are more likely to be vitamin B-6 deficient. Certain autoimmune disorders and some medications also can lead to vitamin B-6 deficiency. For people who lack vitamin B-6, a supplement may be necessary.

 Having the right balance of vitamins and minerals in your body is important for good health. However, getting too much of some nutrients, usually from high-dose supplements, can be dangerous.

Vitamin B-6 may reduce the severity of morning sickness during pregnancy. If you have persistent nausea and vomiting, your pregnancy care team might prescribe vitamin B-6 supplements.

VITAMIN B-12

Vitamin B-12 (cobalamin) plays an essential role in red blood cell formation, cell metabolism, nerve function and the production of DNA inside cells. Food sources of vitamin B-12 include poultry, meat, fish and dairy products. Vitamin B-12 is also added to some foods, such as fortified breakfast cereals, and is available as an oral supplement.

Vitamin B-12 deficiency isn't common in the United States. However, you might consider a vitamin B-12 supplement if you follow a vegetarian or vegan diet, as plant foods don't contain vitamin B-12. Older adults and people with digestive tract conditions that affect absorption of nutrients also are susceptible to vitamin B-12 deficiency and may benefit from a supplement.

VITAMIN C

Vitamin C (ascorbic acid) is a nutrient your body needs to help form blood vessels, cartilage, muscle and collagen. Vitamin C has antioxidant properties and is vital to your body's healing process. It also helps your body absorb and store iron. Your body doesn't naturally produce vitamin C. Most people get enough vitamin C from a healthy diet. Vitamin C is found in citrus fruits, berries, potatoes, tomatoes, peppers, cabbage, Brussels sprouts, broccoli and spinach.

Vitamin C deficiency is more common in people who smoke, who have certain illnesses that disrupt vitamin absorption or who don't regularly eat vegetables and fruits.

If you take vitamin C for its antioxidant properties, keep in mind that the supplement might not offer the same benefits as naturally occurring antioxidants in food.

VITAMIN D

Vitamin D is a nutrient your body needs for building and maintaining healthy bones. That's because your body can absorb calcium, the primary component of bone, only when vitamin D is present. Vitamin D also regulates many other cellular functions in your body. Its anti-inflammatory, antioxidant and neuroprotective properties support immune health, muscle function and brain cell activity.

Your body makes vitamin D when direct sunlight converts a chemical in your skin into an active form of the vitamin (calciferol). Vitamin D isn't

160   Mayo Clinic Guide to Holistic Health

FOOD VS. SUPPLEMENTS

You can get your entire daily requirement of vitamin C by just popping a pill. You can get the same amount by eating a large orange. So which is better? In most cases, the orange is better. Whole foods — such as fruits, vegetables, whole grains and dairy products — have benefits you can't find in a pill, including:

- **Greater nutrition** Whole foods contain a variety of nutrients your body needs, not just one. An orange, for example, provides vitamin C as well as beta carotene, calcium and other nutrients. Vitamin C supplements lack these other nutrients.
- **Essential fiber** Fiber is important for digestion. It also helps prevent certain diseases. For instance, soluble fiber (found in beans, some grains and some fruits and vegetables) and insoluble fiber (found in whole grains and some fruits and vegetables) may help prevent heart disease, diabetes and constipation.
- **Phytochemicals** Many foods — including some fruits, vegetables, whole grains, legumes and nuts — contain naturally occurring food substances called phytochemicals. These substances may help protect you against cancer, heart disease, osteoporosis and diabetes.

naturally found in many foods, but you can get it from fortified milk, fortified cereal and fatty fish such as salmon, mackerel and sardines. If you're concerned that you have little sun exposure or aren't getting enough vitamin D in your diet, talk to a healthcare professional about whether a vitamin supplement might be right for you.

RISKS AND SAFETY CONCERNS

Having the right balance of vitamins and minerals in your body is important for good health. However, getting too much of some nutrients, usually from high-dose supplements, can be dangerous. Here's how to be supplement smart:

- **Know the risks** Some vitamins and minerals can be flushed out of the body easily without serious harm, even if you take too much. But taking high-dose supplements of certain nutrients that can't be easily eliminated can be dangerous. Too much vitamin A can lead to liver failure. Too much vitamin D can affect levels of calcium in the

blood. Overdoing iron can cause digestive system issues and might interfere with absorption of medications.
- **Stay under the limit** A tolerable upper intake level (UL) has been established for many vitamins and minerals. A UL is defined as the highest level of daily intake that is unlikely to cause harmful health effects in most people. This amount includes how much of a nutrient you get from both food and supplements. To be safe, stay under each UL unless specifically advised otherwise.
- **Get a checkup** It's best to get a medical professional's perspective before starting any supplement. Many supplements interfere with medications and even with each other. Bring your bottles so your care team can see the ingredients.
- **Check the labels** The marking "USP Verified" on the label ensures that the product meets strength, quality and purity standards set forth by the U.S. Pharmacopeia, which is an independent testing organization. Watch the expiration date. Vitamins and minerals can become less effective over time.

OUR TAKE

If you eat a variety of foods, including plenty of vegetables and fruits, whole grains, lean proteins and low-fat dairy products, you most likely are getting all the vitamins and minerals you need in the best way possible — from your diet.

Although supplements may not offer all the benefits that whole foods can provide, there are times when taking vitamins and minerals in pill form may be appropriate. For instance, if you don't eat the recommended servings of fruits, vegetables and other healthy foods, you may benefit from a multivitamin that contains a variety of essential nutrients. Multivitamins also can be helpful if you are vegan or vegetarian, eat a diet that's limited because of food allergies or intolerances, or have a disease or condition that doesn't allow you to digest or absorb nutrients properly. Older age and certain lifestyle habits, such as smoking and excessive alcohol consumption, can make it difficult to get all the nutrients you need from food.

As for boosting the amount of specific vitamins and minerals you consume, there are times when this can make sense, especially for women. If you're pregnant or trying to become pregnant, certain nutrients — such as calcium, folic acid and iron — are needed more than ever to protect your health and the health of your developing baby. In addition, supplementing your diet with calcium and vitamin D is often considered crucial following menopause to protect against osteoporosis and the risk of fractures.

Music therapy

On December 14 and 15, 2023, the National Institutes of Health (NIH) hosted a medical workshop unique in the agency's history. Most medical meetings consist of presentations, discussions and the Q&A sessions that follow. Music, especially live music, is rarely heard at such events. But this event was different.

Produced in collaboration with the National Endowment for the Arts, the Renée Fleming Foundation and the John F. Kennedy Center for the Performing Arts, the workshop included multiple live performances. The goal was to demonstrate the power that music has over people and their minds — and present the science behind it. Titled "Music as Medicine: The Science and Clinical Practice," the NIH workshop highlighted the healing powers of music.

HOW MUSIC CAN ENHANCE HEALTH

Music has the power not only to move us but also, research finds, to improve our mood and reduce stress. Instinctively we sense that music can make us feel better; science is identifying the biological underpinnings as to why. Listening to music may help our brain cells process information better and improve our mental and emotional functioning. For example, scientists have learned that listening to music increases blood flow to brain regions that generate and control emotions, such as the brain's limbic system, which kicks into gear when our ears hear music.

Music also may promote the production of feel-good hormones. The chills, goose bumps or other bodily sensations you feel when you listen to a piece of music that moves you deeply may be because your body releases dopamine — a neurotransmitter that triggers sensations of pleasure and well-being. As you become more familiar with a particular song, your body may release dopamine as soon as you hear the song's first notes. Music is also known to have pain-relieving properties, likely because it distracts the brain from focusing on pain and because it causes dopamine release.

Some scientists think that music's effect may be even more direct. They theorize that because sound waves are ultimately vibrations, these vibrations can directly affect neuromuscular structures in the body.

Music has so much power that some nearly noncommunicative people with Alzheimer's disease have sung along when hearing music from their youth. Music evokes strong emotions, and emotions enhance memory processes. Many adults still remember the words from favorite songs from their high school years — in large part because emotions are so strong during adolescence, a time when the brain is rapidly developing.

HOW MUSIC THERAPY WORKS

Because of music's positive effects on well-being, it has been explored as a therapeutic agent. Therapists use music interventions to help people in a variety of settings.

For example, a music therapist may use song and dance to help students with learning disorders find new ways to achieve communication or physical coordination skills. To improve mental health, therapists may play recorded music to bring up emotions and start conversations that help clients process their feelings. Music therapy can help:
- Decrease anxiety
- Decrease blood pressure
- Decrease pain symptoms
- Elevate mood
- Improve quality of life
- Slow heart rate

All styles of music can be helpful in music therapy. Some techniques that music therapists might use include:
- Guided imagery and music
- Improvisation
- Lyric analysis
- Movement to music
- Music-assisted relaxation
- Song writing
- Therapeutic singing

Music therapists are credentialed professionals who train in a variety of subjects including music theory, anatomy and counseling. You can find music therapists in many places, including schools, hospitals, psychiatric facilities, elder care facilities and hospices.

WHAT THE RESEARCH SHOWS

Clinical trials suggest that that music therapy can help ease symptoms and improve function in a variety of conditions, including the following.

Music has so much power that some nearly noncommunicative people with Alzheimer's disease have sung along when hearing music from their youth.

Pain
In a small study of people with fibromyalgia, researchers found that listening to pleasant, relaxing music, chosen individually, significantly reduced pain and increased mobility.

Alzheimer's
When caregivers who assisted people with dementia and Alzheimer's sang for them during their morning care routine, the patients changed their behavior to be more cooperative, present and responsive. One person started to speak in sentences, which she hadn't done for a long time. Another washed her hands without prompting. Yet another looked her caregiver in the eyes and said they were beautiful.

Stroke
One study looked at the effects of music on people who had experienced a stroke. Study participants who listened to music daily experienced better recovery in terms of thinking and verbal memory after two months compared with those who didn't. Their focused attention also improved greatly. Plus the music group was in a better mood and less depressed or confused.

Exercise performance
Another study found that listening to preferred music while exercising can have positive effects on performance, including helping the exerciser run faster and longer. In fact, participants ran at significantly faster speed while listening to music compared to running with no music.

Autism
Research suggests that children with autism tend to respond better to music than they do to spoken words. One small study showed that music therapy can help children with autism improve their social skills. The researchers noted that music therapy encourages children to establish relationships with others and better understand how other people feel.

Cerebral palsy
A review of several studies found that some sounds, whether musical or not — also described as vibroacoustic therapy — produced improvement in motor function in people with cerebral palsy.

RISKS AND SAFETY CONCERNS
There are virtually no risks or safety concerns for enjoying music. Just make sure you are listening at the appropriate volume, as too-loud sounds can damage your hearing.

OUR TAKE
Music therapy has the potential for helping a variety of people with different health needs, with few to no side effects. If music therapy seems like it might be helpful for you or someone you care for, talk to your healthcare team and ask for recommendations. You also can visit the American Music Therapy Association's website (*www.musictherapy.org*) to learn more about music therapy and search for a local music therapist. And of course, feel free to enjoy your favorite music as often as you can.

Naturopathy

Naturopathy is a holistic approach to medicine that blends age-old healing traditions with current research. Its underlying philosophy is that the body has an innate ability to resist disease, recover from illness and self-regulate to keep overall health in balance. Conceptually, these ideas resonate with many notions of traditional Chinese medicine and other holistic health systems.

Modern naturopathy grew out of the healing traditions of the 18th and 19th centuries — although some of its practices have been used much longer than that, dating back to the time of Hippocrates. Early naturopaths often prescribed hydrotherapy — soaks in hot springs, mineral baths and other water-related therapies to promote health.

Today, naturopathic practitioners draw on a combination of many therapies, including modern medicine such as vaccines when appropriate, to treat their patients. Not all naturopathic remedies are supported by scientific evidence. But naturopathy's focus on healthy lifestyle and treating the whole person may have benefits for people with chronic conditions.

BENEFITS OF NATUROPATHY

In embracing the idea that the body can heal itself, naturopathy encourages individuals to strive for optimal wellness by way of lifestyle. This might include diet and exercise recommendations, massage, acupuncture, herbal supplements, heat and cold therapies, and mind-body therapies. When diseases develop, treatments are meant to address the root cause of the underlying condition, rather than just its symptoms.

In doing so, naturopaths begin with minimal interventions and proceed to more robust ones as needed. For example, the first level of defense against illness could be transitioning to a healthier diet and lifestyle. Next could be boosting blood circulation, such as with water therapy. The third step might involve strengthening the body with herbs or specific exercises, such as yoga. The fourth step might use massage or another physical manipulation, and the fifth step would be to loop in dietary supplements. Naturopaths typically resort to using medications or surgery only when these prior steps don't help.

In the United States, naturopathy is practiced by naturopathic physicians, traditional naturopaths and other healthcare professionals who offer naturopathic services.

WHAT NATUROPATHIC PRACTITIONERS DO

Naturopathic practitioners use many different treatment approaches, including:
- Dietary and lifestyle changes
- Stress reduction
- Herbs and other dietary supplements
- Homeopathy
- Manipulative therapies
- Exercise therapy
- Practitioner-guided detoxification
- Psychotherapy and counseling

Some practitioners use other methods as well or, if appropriate, may refer patients to conventional healthcare professionals.

Not all naturopathic practitioners are the same, and not all of them have the same type of education. There are three kinds of naturopathic practitioners: naturopathic physicians, traditional naturopaths and healthcare professionals who practice naturopathy.

- **Naturopathic physicians** complete a four-year, graduate-level program at one of the North American naturopathic medical schools accredited by the Council on Naturopathic Medical Education, which is recognized by the U.S. Department of Education. Some states and territories of the U.S. have licensing requirements for naturopathic physicians and others don't. In the jurisdictions that require licensing, naturopathic physicians must graduate from a four-year naturopathic medical college and pass an examination to receive a license.
- **Traditional naturopaths**, also known simply as "naturopaths," may receive training in a variety of ways. Training programs vary in length and content and are not always accredited by official organizations. Traditional naturopaths are often not eligible for licensing.

A naturopathic physician may be a great partner to guide you to healthy foods, exercise and other wellness practices.

- **Other healthcare professionals** such as physicians, osteopathic doctors, chiropractors, dentists and nurses sometimes offer naturopathic treatments for which they have additional training.

WHAT THE RESEARCH SAYS
Naturopathy hasn't been deeply researched and the studies that exist are small.

Osteoarthritis and rheumatoid arthritis
A small study found that naturopathic interventions including diet, yoga and massage helped people with osteoarthritis and rheumatoid arthritis deal with pain. The interventions also improved quality of life. This study found that women experienced higher treatment satisfaction compared with men.

Risk of heart disease
Another small study found that naturopathic healing reduced the risk of heart disease in people with metabolic syndrome. Metabolic syndrome is a cluster of conditions that occur together, increasing risk of heart disease, stroke and type 2 diabetes. These conditions include high blood pressure, high blood sugar, excess body fat around the waist and abnormal cholesterol or triglyceride levels.

Blood pressure and weight loss
In one research effort, about 100 people with high blood pressure underwent a naturopathic intervention that modified their diet and lifestyle. Participants followed a vegetarian diet, rich in plant proteins, with no added salt or sugar. They also practiced yoga and underwent massages and steam baths. Three months later, many of them had lost weight and their blood pressure had decreased to the point that some were able to reduce or even stop taking medication for high blood pressure.

OUR TAKE

Naturopathy can be a good way to promote health and maintain wellness. A naturopathic physician may be a great partner to guide you to healthy foods, exercise and other wellness practices. Naturopathic physicians also can offer guidance for many minor ailments and illnesses. But in cases of a serious disease or condition, such as a heart attack or cancer, conventional medical treatment is more effective. Naturopathy may offer much in terms of wellness promotion, but your conventional healthcare team is best when it comes to treating and managing medical conditions that require more than self-care.

Pilates

Pilates is a set of exercises that builds core muscle strength and boosts endurance. It's offered in many modern gyms and spas.

As a practice, however, Pilates isn't new. It was developed in the early 20th century by Joseph Pilates, who was born to Greek parents in Germany in 1883. As a child Pilates was sick and frail, battling rheumatic fever, rickets and chronic asthma. As a teenager, increasingly frustrated with his constant poor health, he began to explore ways to heal and grow stronger. His efforts worked spectacularly well: By performing rigorous exercise regimens taken from the ancient Greeks and Romans, Pilates' health and strength improved so much that by the age of 14 he was an accomplished gymnast, boxer and skier — and according to some, a member of a group of Chinese acrobats. In 1912, at the age of 32, he moved to England, where he became a professional boxer and self-defense teacher, counting members of the British police force among his trainees.

When World War I started, Pilates, as a German national, was interned as an "enemy alien" and had to reside in a camp. To stay fit, he and his fellow inmates devised a series of exercises combining physical fitness with mental acuity and control of breathing to build physical strength and flexibility.

Later in the war, while working as a hospital orderly, Pilates observed the plight of disabled and bedridden soldiers trying to heal from battle injuries. He began working with them, sometimes using old hospital bedsprings to provide resistance training for their weakened muscles. In 1920, Pilates moved to New York, where he met his future wife, Clara, one of his first patients with chronic arthritis. When they opened their exercise studio, it was frequented by many famous dancers seeking to build muscle strength and recover from injuries, including Martha Graham, Hanya Holm and George Balanchine.

Today, the term *Pilates* is used to refer to a holistic practice involving gentle movements that engage the mind, body and spirit. Pilates uses a combination of approximately 50 simple, repetitive exercises to boost muscle strength, endurance and flexibility, as well as promote healing from injuries. It's also used to improve posture and balance. The exercises are designed to engage the muscles of the entire body, including the abdominal and pelvic ones.

Pilates exercises can be performed either on a mat or on specialized equipment called a reformer. When using the mat, participants typically sit or lie supine or prone while lifting, moving or holding still legs, arms and their body. On the reformer — a sliding horizontal platform within a box-like frame upon which a person sits, stands, kneels or reclines — muscle-building resistance is provided via light springs attached to the platform and through a pulley system. While Pilates aims to build muscle strength, it won't create bulky muscles. Rather, the intention is to help you achieve a longer, leaner look.

WHAT THE RESEARCH SAYS

Research into the health benefits of Pilates is scarce and often inconclusive. But the practice seems to aid in muscle strength and endurance, as well as provide other holistic health benefits.

Strength, balance and endurance
A systematic review of several studies found that Pilates can improve flexibility, balance and muscular endurance.

One small study of women engaged in Pilates found that the practice improved their abdominal and respiratory muscle strength. Another small study found that when middle-aged men and women practiced Pilates exercise for 12 weeks, for two 60-minute sessions per week, they boosted abdominal and upper-body muscular endurance and increased hamstring strength. But they didn't improve their overall posture.

Back pain
A meta-analysis found that Pilates may help relieve discomfort in people with chronic low back pain.

Mental health
A small study found that practicing Pilates for an hour once a week for 10 weeks had physical and psychological benefits, including better mood. A systematic review found that Pilates exercises lessened the severity of depression symptoms in women.

Pilates can be effective in improving muscle strength, endurance, flexibility, balance and mood. It also may help you recover from injuries.

Scoliosis
One review effort suggested that Pilates exercises may help with scoliosis — a curvature of the spine. The review found that Pilates exercises can be applied to reduce asymmetrical posture in people with mild scoliosis, but that overall, the evidence is limited.

Stroke
A review of several studies found moderate evidence that Pilates improved balance in people recovering from stroke.

FINDING A PILATES INSTRUCTOR
There's no license required to teach Pilates. If you're doing Pilates to address a particular health concern, look for an instructor with proper training in Pilates techniques and experience teaching people with conditions like yours. You might also ask your healthcare team for recommendations.

RISKS AND SAFETY CONCERNS
In some cases, Pilates can make certain health conditions worse. Talk to your healthcare team before engaging in Pilates if you have any of the following:
- Herniated and bulging spine discs.
- Spine instability, a condition in which vertebrae move more than they should.
- Spinal stenosis, a narrowing of the spinal canal or nerve root canals.
- Hypermobility, a condition in which joints move beyond the usual range.
- Osteoporosis, a disease characterized by deterioration of bone tissue.

When properly applied, Pilates may help improve some of these conditions, but it must be used with caution and after a consultation with your healthcare team.

OUR TAKE
Pilates can be effective in improving muscle strength, endurance, flexibility, balance and mood. It also may help you recover from injuries. It can be an easy exercise routine to adhere to and may even help with some forms of back pain. However, there are some circumstances where it would be wise to talk to your healthcare team before starting a Pilates practice (see above).

Probiotics

Probiotics are popular dietary supplements commonly touted as a remedy for numerous intestinal and other conditions. Is this just another fad or do they indeed provide tangible benefits? It depends on exactly what's in them, but the aim is to improve your health by changing the bacteria in your digestive tract, also called your gut. The term *probiotics*, derived from a Greek word meaning "for life," refers to friendly living microorganisms that contribute beneficially to their host.

FRIENDLY BACTERIA

Your gut contains trillions of bacteria, which play an important role in your body. They help you digest food, breaking it down into compounds that can be absorbed by the lining in your stomach. They synthesize a variety of vitamins and amino acids — the basic building blocks of all proteins produced by your body. And they also protect you from harmful bacteria that may sneak into your intestine from the environment.

Your gut microbes are territorial, a feature that can be beneficial. Not only do microorganisms colonize your gut to prevent foreign species from taking hold but they also produce antimicrobial compounds that destroy the invaders. Moreover, recent studies found that gut microbes also can directly talk to the immune system — by way of biochemical messaging — and mediate its response to harmful germs. Cumulatively, these microscopic bodyguards are known as your gut microbiome.

Probiotics are foods or supplements that contain such beneficial bacteria. The science of probiotics may sound novel, but it's been over 100 years in the making. In the early 20th century, Russian microbiologist Ilya Metchnikov, who spent most of his career working at the Louis Pasteur Institute in Paris and who won a Nobel Prize in immunology, proclaimed that intestinal microbes play a key role in human health.

At the time, cholera epidemics were common but the disease affected individuals differently. In the same household, some people might die, while others might be only mildly sick or not at all. Metchnikov hypothesized that those who didn't succumb to cholera carried microbes in their stomachs that fought off the disease. Over a century later, science confirmed that he was right — some people who live in areas where cholera was or still is common harbor specific bacteria that keep cholera at bay.

Metchnikov also laid the foundation for probiotics and the science of longevity. While studying centenarians living in Eastern Europe, he noticed that their diet included a lot of yogurt, a food that's typically full of probiotic bacteria. Metchnikov theorized that yogurt helped maintain healthy gut bacteria and hold off the diseases of aging.

Today, science is finding that the gut microbiome is indeed linked in important ways to health. Moreover, scientists now know that beneficial bacteria live in other places on the body, such as the skin, throat and nose.

Fermented foods such as yogurt have been viewed as beneficial to health throughout history. Many ancient cultures used fermented milk as part of their daily diets, including Egyptians, Mongols and Europeans. Some sources even claim that the Hebrew patriarch Abraham owed his longevity to fermented milk.

SYMBIOSIS AND DYSBIOSIS

There are many different probiotic bacterial strains, but some of the most common ones that dwell in the human gut belong to groups called *Lactobacillus* and *Bifidobacterium*. A few other types of bacteria also may be probiotics, and so may some yeasts such as *Saccharomyces boulardii*. Fermented foods such as sauerkraut and kombucha also contain probiotics.

Besides probiotics, there are also prebiotics, which are substances that stimulate the growth of probiotic bacteria. For example, dietary fiber is a prebiotic. While humans don't digest fiber directly, gut microbes do

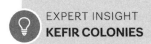

EXPERT INSIGHT
KEFIR COLONIES

Ask Ryan T. Hurt, M.D., Ph.D., a specialist in clinical nutrition and management of complex medical conditions, why he keeps an empty bottle of kefir in his office and he might tell you it's the medical tool he uses to talk to patients about the benefits of probiotics. "There are 56 billion colonies per cup," he says of the number of beneficial bacteria thriving in the drink. "When you ingest them, they settle in your intestines, doing what they normally do — digesting food and warding off invaders."

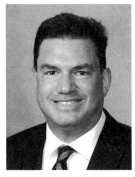

Ryan T. Hurt, M.D., Ph.D.
General Internal Medicine

feed on it, which boosts their numbers. When you combine prebiotics and probiotics, you get symbiosis. "I usually recommend pre- and probiotics," says Mayo Clinic internist Ryan T. Hurt, M.D., Ph.D., because "there's clear data emerging now that when you combine them, you get the best results."

When the microbes in your gut are properly balanced, they are symbiotic to you, Dr. Hurt explains. Your digestive system is working well, your body is extracting nutrients from the food, you have energy to go about your daily life and your immune system is strong. But certain factors — such as infections, unhealthy diets or antibiotic overuse — can mess up this balance and create dysbiosis, a state in which some microbial populations get out of control. "There's symbiosis and there's dysbiosis," explains Dr. Hurt. "Dysbiosis is an abnormal increase of the overall bacterial population, but also particular bacteria that are going to cause more symptoms."

A gut that is rich in healthy bacteria may help reduce the risk of inflammatory illnesses such as inflammatory bowel disease, irritable bowel syndrome, obesity and colon cancer. Microbiome imbalances, on the other hand, can lead to digestive problems, metabolic disorders and inflammatory conditions such as Crohn's disease and ulcerative colitis.

Overuse of antibiotics can cause conditions such as small intestine bacterial overgrowth or SIBO, in which certain bacterial populations balloon out of proportion, causing digestive problems that can severely affect quality of life and in some cases become life-threatening. Antibiotics that are too strong can wipe out normal gut dwellers, which allows more aggressive and unhealthy species, such as *Clostridioides difficile*, to take hold. An overgrowth of *C. difficile* causes recurring bouts of diarrhea and is difficult to treat.

More recently, gut dysbiosis has been linked to a slew of health conditions, including depression, anxiety, bipolar disorders, autism, schizophrenia, Parkinson's disease, Alzheimer's disease, dementia, multiple sclerosis and even epilepsy.

GETTING TO GUT HARMONY

Can dysbiosis be fixed? And how can the symbiotic state be maintained? There's a lot of research looking into these questions, but exactly which bacteria you should be ingesting and how much remain in question.

For starters, scientists don't yet know exactly what constitutes a healthy microbiome. Moreover, the concept of a healthy microbiome may differ depending on your age, genetics, diet and even where you live and with whom. "The microbiome is influenced by a lot of things, whether it be the animals and pets you live with, where you live and whom you're living with," says Dr. Hurt. "You're incorporating different pieces of their microbiome into yours."

Establishing the proper probiotic and prebiotic doses is also challenging. Unlike vitamins or medicines, bacteria are living organisms. They may multiply inside the intestine — or some of them may die out. And they may or may not play well with other bacterial species in the gut.

That's why your best bet is getting your probiotics and prebiotics in food form, says Dr. Hurt. It's also the most holistic and natural way. Probiotics are commonly found in fermented foods, including:

- Buttermilk
- Kefir
- Kimchi
- Kombucha
- Miso
- Sauerkraut
- Sourdough
- Tempeh
- Yogurt with live cultures
- Fermented vegetables

Prebiotic fiber can be derived from:

- Fruits
- Vegetables
- Legumes
- Grains

If you choose to use probiotic supplements, do a bit of research before deciding on a brand. A good probiotic must meet several criteria, including the following:

- The strains of bacteria listed on a bottle must be the typical dwellers of the human gut.
- They must be clinically demonstrated to offer benefits.
- They must be safe.

It's best if the probiotic contains different strains of bacteria because diversity is beneficial. If you're not sure what probiotics to choose, talk to your healthcare team.

WHAT THE RESEARCH SAYS

Although probiotics are a hot research topic, much remains to be learned about whether they're helpful for various health conditions and how safe they are for people to ingest. Most available studies center around conditions involving the gastrointestinal system. Here's what researchers have found so far.

Diarrhea
Probiotics may help prevent diarrhea caused by *C. difficile* as well as antibiotic-associated diarrhea. A systematic review of more than 20 randomized controlled trials enrolling more than 8,000 people found fairly good evidence that probiotics were effective in preventing diarrhea caused by *C. difficile*. Another systematic review and meta-analysis suggested that probiotics helped reduce antibiotic-associated diarrhea, but more research into the topic is needed.

Ulcerative colitis
Evidence suggests that probiotics have been helpful in improving ulcerative colitis, another hard-to-treat inflammatory condition.

Children's health
Probiotics may be helpful for infants and children. They've shown promise for treatment of infant colic and for prevention of necrotizing enterocolitis, a dangerous condition that affects some premature infants.

One study investigated the use of probiotics for children with acute gastroenteritis — an inflammation of the lining of the stomach and intestine. The children treated with probiotics experienced less diarrhea and spent less time in the hospital than those who didn't use probiotics. However, the study added that the certainty of evidence was very low.

Microplastics
A very recent study found yet another beneficial promise of probiotic bacteria: They seem to help clear the body of heavy metals and microplastics — the tiny plastic particles that leach into our drinking water from the environment and into our meals from food packaging. These microplastics can cause gut inflammation and dysbiosis. The study found that some probiotic bacteria can bind to microplastics and even degrade certain kinds, preventing their damaging effects. But more research is needed to understand these interactions better.

RISKS AND SAFETY CONCERNS
Probiotics have an extensive history of apparently safe use, particularly in healthy people. However, they may not be safe for people with severe illnesses or compromised immune systems. Cases of severe or fatal infections have been reported in premature infants who were given probiotics, and the U.S. Food and Drug Administration has warned healthcare professionals about this risk.

Additionally, some probiotic products have been reported to contain microorganisms other than those listed on the label. In some instances, these contaminants may pose serious health risks. With that said, the side effects of probiotics are generally rare, and most healthy adults can safely add foods that contain prebiotics and probiotics to their diets.

OUR TAKE

Probiotics and prebiotics may play an important role in your overall health — from digestion to metabolism to healthy aging. Mayo Clinic researchers are working on answering further questions, including:
- What can the microbiome reveal about health?
- Can microbial communities in the colon be the cause of irritable bowel symptoms?
- How do gut microbes affect other parts of the body, such as the brain, joints, liver and immune system?
- Can gut microbial metabolites be the reason that diet influences colon cancer development?
- Can genomic sequencing techniques help researchers identify organisms that cause vaginosis and reproductive health problems?
- Can an imbalance in the microbiome lead to autoimmune diseases?
- How do scientists and clinicians translate their insights about the microbiome into new diagnostic and prognostic approaches?

While there are many probiotic supplements available in stores and online, the healthiest and most holistic way of cultivating a healthy gut microbiome is through fermented foods that contain probiotics and fiber-rich foods that act as prebiotics. Talk to your healthcare team to see what probiotics are best for you.

Progressive muscle relaxation

Progressive muscle relaxation is designed to reduce the tension in your muscles and to help reduce stress. You practice it by slowly tensing and then relaxing each muscle group. This can help you focus on the difference between muscle tension and relaxation. You can become more aware of physical sensations and how to help yourself relax and become less tense.

Notably, stress causes more than just muscle tension. It also triggers other physiological responses such as increased heart rate, palpitations, shortness of breath and sweating. Progressively relaxing your whole body can help alleviate these symptoms too. Relaxation techniques slow down your breathing, heart rate and blood pressure. The advantage of this relaxation technique is that it can be used in any setting with only a basic set of instructions and a quiet, comfortable environment.

The idea of progressive muscle relaxation was first set forth by Edmund Jacobson, an American physician who believed that freeing the body of muscular tension could reduce anxiety. He described this method of stress reduction in his book *Progressive Relaxation*, published in 1938.

Progressive relaxation is achieved through tensing and then relaxing various muscle groups in sequence. By doing so, it's possible to identify where extra stress or tension is being stored in the body and then deliberately relieve that tension.

HOW TO DO IT
Choose a quiet, comfortable area where you can lay your body flat. Start by tensing and relaxing the muscles in your toes, then your ankles, calves, thighs and so forth. Progressively work your way up to your neck and head. You also can start with your head and neck and work down to your toes. Check the muscle tension in your face too — wrinkle your forehead, scrunch your eyes (remove contact lenses first), smile as wide as you can and finally press your lips together. Tense each group of muscles for about five seconds, then fully relax those muscles for 30 seconds and repeat.

WHAT THE RESEARCH SAYS
While no major studies have been done on progressive muscle relaxation, there is some evidence that it can help in the treatment of certain conditions. Here are some examples.

Anxiety

In a small study, 10 women between 60 and 84 years old who had lost their husbands within the past five years took part in a five-month progressive relaxation study. The women all felt anxious and tense. After 10 weeks of practicing progressive relaxation, the women all said they felt less anxious.

Stress

In a study conducted several years ago, about 70 men were exposed to a stressful situation. Some men did progressive muscle relaxation. Others listened to classical music, or listened to a story and wrote down what they heard, or simply sat in silence. The men who did progressive relaxation were the most relaxed of all the men in the study and felt the least amount of tension. These men also had lower levels of the stress hormone cortisol in their systems.

Cancer

Studies of women with breast cancer show that progressive muscle relaxation can help reduce nausea, vomiting, anxiety, depression and even how long women have to stay in the hospital after mastectomy.

Another study, which focused on people undergoing surgery for colorectal cancer, found that those who practiced progressive muscle relaxation experienced less anxiety and needed smaller amounts of opioid painkillers than those who did not.

In yet another research effort, progressive muscle relaxation reduced levels of fatigue, anxiety, pain and depression in postsurgical cancer patients, and also helped them sleep better.

High blood pressure

In several clinical studies, relaxation techniques have been shown to lower blood pressure in people with high blood pressure. However, sometimes studies used different types of relaxation therapies or relaxation was paired with other therapies, which makes it difficult to tell

Progressive muscle relaxation can be done just about anywhere and can reduce stress, ease tension and clear the mind within a few minutes.

exactly how helpful progressive muscle relaxation techniques are. Still, progressive muscle relaxation does appear to be linked to a reduction in blood pressure.

Headache

One study found that after learning progressive relaxation techniques, people experiencing migraine had substantially fewer migraine headaches.

OUR TAKE

Anyone experiencing stress can benefit from progressive muscle relaxation. A big plus of progressive muscle relaxation technique is that it's easy to do. It can be especially helpful for beginners or people who are new to the idea of using relaxation strategies. It can be done just about anywhere and can reduce stress, ease tension and clear the mind within a few minutes. It's a tool that you can use after a difficult meeting, to unwind at the end of the day or to improve symptoms of a difficult-to-treat condition.

You might decide to use muscle relaxation by itself or combine it with another mind-body approach, such as guided imagery, meditation or music for an even greater effect. Many hospitals and clinics offer relaxation training programs that include progressive muscle relaxation as a holistic way to improve wellness.

Psychedelics

Many people associate the term *psychedelics* with illicit drugs that are best avoided. There's definite truth in that — substances such as LSD and magic mushrooms can create an altered sense of time and space and distorted perceptions of the environment. They also can cause psychotic symptoms, confusion and dissociation from reality. For these reasons, the 1971 United Nations Convention on Psychotropic Substances restricted the clinical use of these substances, labeling them as drugs of abuse.

Yet with or without regulation, psychedelics have been around for many thousands of years (see opposite page). Most recently they've attracted interest among researchers not as recreational drugs but as medical treatments for mental illness. Scientists are looking into potentially beneficial effects of administering these substances in proper amounts, in controlled settings and for specific conditions.

Many psychedelics are naturally occurring substances in plants from different parts of the world:

- Psilocybin and psilocin are found in about 180 species of mushrooms, such as *Psilocybe cubensis.*
- DMT, which stands for N-dimethyltryptamine, is an active ingredient in ayahuasca, a plant-based Amazonian medicinal drink.
- Mescaline, a naturally occurring cousin of LSD, comes from the peyote cactus.
- Muscimol is found in *Amanita muscaria* mushrooms.
- Ibotenic acid is found in *Amanita pantherina* mushrooms.

Why are these once-discredited compounds back at the scientific forefront? One reason is that effective treatments for severe mental illnesses remain elusive. Despite the wide use of legally available antidepressants, such as the commonly prescribed selective serotonin reuptake inhibitors (SSRIs), depression rates have yet to decline in a meaningful way. On the contrary, in the 21st century in the U.S., rates of depression and mental illness have risen. So have deaths due to suicide, drug overdose and alcohol use disorder.

Another reason is that scientists have built a better understanding of how these substances work on the brain. For example, research has shown that psychedelics increase blood flow to certain brain regions. Also, the way that some psychedelics activate serotonin receptors — which are like gateways for feel-good chemicals in the brain — reduces the energy needed for the brain to switch between different activity states.

> **? DID YOU KNOW?**
>
> The history of using psychedelics is as old as humankind. According to some, the use of psychoactive substances was so widespread in the ancient world as to be considered the norm.
>
> Archaeologists excavating a cave in Bolivia recently found a thousand-year-old ritual bundle belonging to a shaman from the pre-Inca era. Scrapings from the bundle contained traces of several psychotropic compounds, including a metabolite of cocaine, the psychedelic tea known as ayahuasca and psilocin, the active agent in certain psychotropic mushrooms.
>
> Similar compounds have been used by many other ancient cultures. Hunter-gatherer societies across the globe — in the Americas, Eurasia, Australia and Africa — have used them, typically in various religious ceremonies. Greek historian Herodotus wrote about the ritual use of cannabis by the Scythians of the Pontic Steppe. The ancient Greeks and later the ancient Romans held seasonal religious rites that included ritual ingestion of a psychoactive drink called *kykeon* which may have included fungi containing LSD-like compounds. An ancient civilization of Zoroastrians who lived in today's Iran used a similar drink called *haoma*.

As a result, a number of clinical trials have begun for specific psychedelic drugs, such as MDMA, ketamine, LSD, psilocybin and DMT. The growing body of research has so far found psychedelics helpful in treating depression, substance use disorders and anxiety in people with terminal cancer. Research efforts looking into using psychedelics for addiction and post-traumatic stress disorder (PTSD) also have found promising results. Newer studies are investigating psychedelics as possible treatments for migraine and cluster headaches, eating disorders and early dementia.

WHAT THE RESEARCH SAYS
Interest in researching psychedelics is growing and clinical trials are ongoing. In some cases, certain psychedelic substances have shown promise in improving hard-to-treat psychiatric disorders. For example, it's possible that MDMA, more commonly known as ecstasy, may be useful for treating certain mental conditions, but more research is needed.

Addiction

A preliminary study of ayahuasca suggested it might be an effective treatment for addiction to substances such as alcohol, tobacco and cocaine.

Offered as an intervention for the Coast Salish First Nations community in British Columbia, ayahuasca led to significant improvements in mental health and reductions in self-reported use of these substances after six months, with no lasting physical or psychological side effects.

A study of Brazilian religious groups who regularly drink ayahuasca as part of a sacrament indicates that long-term drinkers of ayahuasca tend to have a lower prevalence of substance use compared to people who don't drink it regularly.

Post-traumatic stress disorder

Several research efforts investigated using MDMA for chronic treatment-resistant post-traumatic stress disorder. Compared with current PTSD treatment options, which often involve antidepressants, supervised use of MDMA appears to be safe and effective with long-lasting benefits — possibly superior to current treatments.

In a small pilot trial, researchers found that 20 participants with chronic PTSD — average duration of PTSD was close to 20 years — fared better on experimental MDMA treatment than on currently approved medications. Participants received psychotherapy along with MDMA under the guidance of health professionals and experienced sustained reduction in PTSD symptoms without serious side effects.

Another study investigating MDMA as a treatment for PTSD published similar results — it reduced disease symptoms with few harmful effects. The study concluded that MDMA psychotherapy can be safely administered in a supervised setting with professionals present who are trained to help users navigate the experience and handle potential negative reactions (see "Risks and side effects" on opposite page). Another

Preliminary findings show promise for psychedelics as treatment for pervasive, severe, hard-to-treat psychiatric conditions. But until more studies are done, it is too early to make recommendations on their safety and effectiveness.

study noted that MDMA decreases responses to negative stimuli while increasing trust, empathy and response to social cues and touch.

Depression and anxiety

Preliminary research has shown some effectiveness of psychedelics such as psilocybin, combined with supportive psychotherapy, for treating depression and anxiety. Benefits are more immediate than those obtained with traditional antidepressants, which often take several weeks to show benefit, and often come with fewer side effects.

Some of the difficulty in prescribing psilocybin for a condition such as depression, however, lies in how the treatment is administered. Unlike taking an oral antidepressant at home, a drug like psilocybin must be taken in a clinical setting under the care of professionals trained to monitor safety and provide support before, during and after administration. Such logistical challenges will likely need to be addressed and fine-tuned before adoption of psychedelic treatments can become more widespread.

RISKS AND SAFETY CONCERNS

Although psychedelics are relatively safe physiologically — they don't lead to addiction — in some people they can cause overwhelming distress, commonly described as "a bad trip." This may manifest as acute anxiety, fear, increased heart rate and elevated blood pressure. Without supervision, such symptoms can lead to dangerous behaviors. In some people, certain psychedelics also may cause headaches. While most immediate side effects can be easily managed and don't tend to result in long-term harm, their intensity varies from person to person and must be taken seriously.

OUR TAKE

Medical interest in psychedelics has the potential to change the current treatment approach to mental illness. Preliminary findings show promise for psychedelics as treatment for pervasive, severe, hard-to-treat psychiatric conditions. But until more studies are done, it is too early to make recommendations on their safety and effectiveness. Moreover, the effects of psychedelics vary between people and depend on a person's current emotions and surroundings as well as the dose, so it's important that administration is closely monitored by medical professionals. Using psychedelics at home with no supervision is potentially harmful and is not recommended.

PSYCHEDELICS | Therapies A–Z   **185**

Qigong

Qigong is a mind-body practice that was developed over 5,000 years ago, as part of traditional Chinese medicine. The term *qigong* translates as "cultivating qi" (CHEE), the life energy believed by practitioners of traditional Chinese medicine to flow through the channels inside the human body, nourishing its organs and tissues. When the flow of qi is blocked and it can't reach the organs, health ailments develop. An old Chinese saying states that "qi is the root of a human being," so when qi is weak or imbalanced, diseases take hold. In traditional Chinese medicine, everything in the universe results from the movement and changes of qi, so regulating qi is the key to health.

Qigong aims to normalize and facilitate the flow of qi through the body to improve health, support well-being and treat medical conditions. It is an exercise and meditation system that works to harmonize the body, mind and spirit. Once an ancient Chinese practice, it is now enjoyed by people all over the world. There are multiple forms of qigong, but they all typically focus on mindfulness and self-regulation. A typical qigong session involves meditation, coordinated slow flowing movement and deep rhythmic breathing.

Qi cultivation is performed in a relaxed standing, sitting or lying position. Once ready, the person begins to regulate breathing in concert with specific mental and physical exercises. For example, one form of qigong involves visualizing the energy flowing through the body in synchrony with breathing. After some training, the person begins to feel the qi traveling along the channels. In traditional Chinese medicine it is believed that the mind guides the qi to a specific area of the body and the qi brings the blood with it, improving circulation and leading to good health. The exercises also can improve balance and muscle strength and alleviate chronic pain.

There are literally thousands of qigong styles, but these three are taught most often:
- The Eight Brocades
- The Six Healing Sounds
- The Five Animal Frolics

Qigong can be practiced for as little as a few minutes or for as much as half an hour or longer. The best time to practice is considered to be when the sun is rising in the morning. That's when the yang energy is thought to be active and fast-moving, which helps jump-start the day. In the evening you might choose to practice calming movements to unwind from a tense or stressful day.

HOW TO FIND A QUALIFIED PRACTITIONER

Qigong instructors don't need a license. There's no national standard for qigong certification. Various qigong organizations offer training and certification programs, with differing criteria and certification levels. When considering taking a qigong class or joining a group, ask the teacher what type of certification they have, ask what to expect from the class, and inform them of your goals and health status.

WHAT THE RESEARCH SHOWS

Current research suggests qigong may improve balance, pain management, strength, brain function, sleep, immune system activity and breathing capacity.

Chronic fatigue
One study suggested qigong as a possible standalone therapy for chronic fatigue syndrome.

Mobility and balance
Another study found that qigong was effective in improving mobility and balance in older adults.

Parkinson's disease
A meta-analysis supported qigong as an alternative therapy to improve walking ability, motor function and balance for patients with Parkinson's disease.

Strength and posture
One small study found that a 12-week qigong exercise program was beneficial for muscle strength and posture control in middle-aged and older women.

There's a small yet growing body of evidence that qigong can improve balance, pain management, brain function, sleep and breathing capacity.

Memory and cognition

Two separate multi-study reviews suggested that qigong may improve memory and thinking processes, also called cognition. The benefits accumulated over time — after 3 to 6 months of regular sessions several times a week in this case. How long the benefits lasted remained unclear, as researchers didn't follow up with participants after the studies ended.

EXPERT INSIGHT
THE SCIENCE OF QI

In Western culture, the concept of cultivating life energy may seem a bit unusual, but Alexander Do, L.Ac., an acupuncturist at Mayo Clinic and a qigong practitioner, has an explanation. Qi is the breath of life that embraces all manifestations of bioenergy, from weather patterns to movement, thought, emotions, and nerve impulses, he explains. In the Chinese language, the character for *qi* is depicted as rice being cooked, creating vapors. It also can mean air or oxygen. "So, through the scientific lens, we can view it as cellular respiration that creates energy to fuel our cells," Do says. "From that perspective, abundant qi takes its origin in good nutrition, oxygen, rest and activity. Efficient bodies can help optimize our health and age gracefully." Cultivating qi helps us get there.

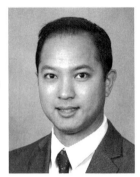

Alexander Do, L.Ac.
Integrative Medicine and Health

Another important concept in traditional Chinese medicine are the two opposing forces called yin and yang. When the yin and yang are balanced, qi can be cultivated and flow well. "The qigong exercises follow the principles of the yin and yang, which means that the world is balanced through polar opposites," Do says. "Therefore, an excess of anything can lead to imbalance, resulting in illness. If the yin and yang are balanced, qi can be cultivated and free-flowing. Qigong practices are ideal for health and healing, as the goal is to harmonize our bodies internally and externally."

Do also practices tai chi, a type of qigong and a form of Chinese martial art. Read more about Do's insights on tai chi on page 211.

RISKS AND SAFETY CONCERNS

Qigong appears to be a safe physical activity. Evidence indicates few, if any, side effects in people practicing qigong, including older adults and people with chronic diseases. A review of studies of adults with neck pain found that qigong and other exercises had similar side effects, which occurred in less than 10% of the participants and included muscle pain, soreness and headache.

There is no research on the safety of qigong during pregnancy and extremely limited research on practicing qigong while pregnant. If you're pregant, talk to your healthcare team before starting qigong. You may need to avoid or modify some qigong movements.

That said, a small 2010 study of 70 healthy pregnant women in Korea found that adding a qigong-like practice to routine prenatal care resulted in several benefits: greater mother-child bonding before birth, fewer maternal depressive symptoms and reduced maternal physical discomfort. The intervention, called qi exercise, involved meditation, breathing and various stretching, strengthening and balancing exercises done while standing, sitting, or lying down. The women experienced no harmful effects.

OUR TAKE

There's a small yet growing body of evidence that qigong can improve balance, pain management, brain function, sleep and breathing capacity. According to a recent survey of tai chi and qigong use among U.S. adults, Americans' engagement in these practices grew 64% from 2007 to 2017. Because there's little or no cost associated with it — you can practice alone or with a group of friends — it can be a convenient and inexpensive way to help restore and promote health. That makes it a useful, easy and cost-effective way to exercise.

For beginners, qigong almost always focuses on correcting one's posture, calming the mind and using the breath to guide movements, so there are no downsides. "My advice is to be patient with the results and try it," says Do. "Like anything in life, once we become familiar with something, it can be enjoyable."

Reflexology

Most people would likely enjoy a foot massage — if nothing else, it relaxes and stimulates the muscles after a long day. But there is growing evidence that foot massage — when performed according to a certain set of rules — can offer more than a relaxing experience.

Called reflexology, this holistic therapy focuses on the application of pressure mainly on the feet, but in some cases also on the hands and ears.

Like many other holistic approaches, reflexology is an ancient therapy used for healing purposes by the Chinese, Egyptians and North American indigenous peoples.

The oldest documentation of reflexology usage is found in an Egyptian papyrus depicting medical practitioners treating the hands and feet of their patients. The modern form of reflexology was developed in the late 19th to early 20th century by physical therapist Eunice Ingham and physician William Fitzgerald.

The theory behind reflexology is that specific areas on the soles of your feet and on your hands correspond to other parts of your body, such as your head, neck or internal organs. In that way, your feet and hands serve as a chart for your entire body.

"We usually describe it to people as a map of your internal organs and spine," says Jennifer Hauschulz, a massage therapist at Mayo Clinic Integrative Medicine and Health.

Reflexologists use these maps to guide them. They apply varying amounts of manual pressure to specific areas of the feet to alleviate a problem in the corresponding area or organ in the body. There are two internationally recognized reflexology methods: the Ingham method and

Reflexology appears to have positive effects, alleviating symptoms in a range of conditions. But there isn't a lot of scientific evidence to indicate that the therapy can treat diseases or symptoms.

the Rwo Shur method. The Ingham method is performed without any tools, while the Rwo Shur method uses tools such as wooden sticks.

Proponents of reflexology believe that it provides four main types of health benefits:

- It promotes relaxation and alleviates stress.
- It enhances circulation.
- It assists the body in normalizing metabolism.
- It complements all other healing approaches.

Some of the reasons people choose reflexology are:

- It doesn't use any drugs or chemicals.
- It relaxes the hands and feet as well as the whole body.
- It stimulates the body to release its own pain-relieving compounds.
- It triggers the release of endorphins, the body's "feel-good" chemicals, helping relieve pain by boosting the sense of well-being.
- It promotes recovery from physical injury, especially for the hands and feet.

WHAT THE RESEARCH SAYS

Research into reflexology has grown in recent years, but study results are often inconclusive. Still, several studies funded by the National Cancer Institute and the National Institutes of Health have found that reflexology may reduce pain, anxiety and depression and may enhance relaxation and

REFLEXOLOGY AT MAYO CLINIC

Many Mayo Clinic massage therapists have reflexology certifications and offer it as a service to patients. "It is particularly helpful for patients recovering from abdominal surgeries or those having digestive issues after a surgery," says Jennifer Hauschulz, a Mayo massage therapist. "In those cases, reflexology is really helpful to try to stimulate their digestive systems before they leave the hospital."

So even when the rest of your body is sore, you still can apply pressure to the feet to stimulate the organs. "For example, the intestinal area is located on your sole, near the arch of the foot," says Hauschulz. "And for the headaches, we would be working with points near and along the toes that correspond with sinuses, eyes, neck and ears."

sleep. Some studies have found it to be an effective therapy for strokes, insomnia, asthma, diabetes, premenstrual syndrome, dementia, cancers and multiple sclerosis.

Cancer pain
Several studies suggest that reflexology, sometimes as brief as five minutes per foot, helped alleviate cancer- and chemotherapy-related symptoms, including pain and nausea, and promoted relaxation.

Multiple sclerosis
One study found reflexology to be moderately effective at easing fatigue and depression and improving overall quality of life in people with multiple sclerosis.

Mental health
A meta-analysis of 26 studies found reflexology to be an effective treatment for depression, anxiety and sleep problems.

Childbirth
Several small studies have found that reflexology helps alleviate labor pain. One study found that women recovering from cesarean childbirth experienced less pain after foot massage and asked for fewer painkillers.

Another small study found that when nurses provided foot reflexology to women at a postpartum care center, it helped alleviate fatigue, stress and depression.

OUR TAKE
On the surface, reflexology appears to have positive effects, alleviating symptoms in a range of conditions. There's little risk involved in reflexology, and massaging the soles of your feet can feel good. But there isn't a lot of scientific evidence to indicate that the therapy can treat various diseases or symptoms. While evidence that reflexology may provide symptomatic relief for various conditions is growing, many studies demonstrate inconclusive results. This indicates that more research is needed.

Reiki

The term *Reiki* (RAY-kee) is made up of the Japanese words *rei*, which means "universal spirit," and *ki*, which (like qi) means "life force energy that nourishes all living beings."

As with other energy therapies, people who specialize in Reiki believe that disturbances in the body's energy systems can cause illness, and that by improving the flow and balance of energy, disease can be treated and overall health maintained. Reiki evolved from ancient Tibetan Buddhist teachings and was popularized by Japanese monk Mikao Usui in the early 1920s.

Today Reiki is used in hospitals, medical centers, hospices and private practice as a holistic approach to healing and well-being. It is believed that Reiki can help with a wide range of conditions that can be difficult to treat with conventional approaches, including migraine, asthma, anxiety, depression, insomnia and chronic fatigue.

Reiki-trained practitioners use their hands or light touch to support and promote the health and healing of the people they treat. With Reiki, these noninvasive hand techniques aim to balance the human energy field as well as surrounding energy fields. The goal is to restore harmony in the energy system and promote relaxation, thus giving the person the opportunity to heal.

The practitioner holds their hands either on or a few inches above the recipient's body in several specific places that may correspond to chakras — the body's spiritual or energy centers — moving from head to toe. Each position may be held for a few minutes. Reiki is commonly used to address stress, pain, anxiety, fatigue and nausea from chemotherapy, and to induce relaxation and enhance well-being.

> There's some evidence that Reiki helps with pain, fatigue and anxiety. And some research suggests that Reiki could have beneficial effects on blood pressure and heart rate. But more study is needed for a definitive conclusion.

Reiki practitioners can achieve three different levels of training.

- **Level One** focuses on learning Reiki for self-care and for delivering it to others in person, by placing your hands either on or above their body. It is taught by a Reiki master and involves so-called *attunement*, which "opens up" the person to *ki*, the universal energy.
- **Level Two** involves learning how to use Reiki from a distance so it can be delivered remotely. It involves a next-level attunement process.
- **Level Three** is considered Reiki master training, which equips the person with the ability to teach Reiki and administer attunement to others.

WHAT TO EXPECT DURING A REIKI SESSION

During a Reiki session, which typically lasts 30 to 60 minutes, you sit or lie down fully clothed while the practitioner holds their hands over the chakras or energy centers on your body.

Recipients often describe a deep sense of relaxation during and after a session, accompanied by a feeling of well-being, which tends to last after the session is over. They also report sensations of warmth, tingling and sleepiness, and feelings of refreshment.

Reiki affects each person differently, so exactly what you will feel is hard to predict. For some people, their symptoms ease and they experience less pain or nausea. Others may sleep better after a session. "Everyone has an individual response to Reiki, so we like to encourage people to not really have any expectations and to just be open to how it will work for them," says Susanne M. Cutshall, a clinical nurse specialist and Reiki practitioner at Mayo Clinic.

FINDING A QUALIFIED PRACTITIONER

There's no official accreditation for Reiki specialists, but there are several organizations that may be helpful for finding a qualified practitioner. The International Reiki Organization (*www.reikiassociation.com*) offers an online search function for qualified local practitioners. It also provides training opportunities for people interested in learning Reiki. The International Reiki Association (*www.iarp.org*) helps those new to Reiki learn how to use it or become a master. Some universities are now offering Reiki education and courses. The University of Minnesota Center for Spirituality and Healing (*https://csh.umn.edu*) offers such opportunities.

Because Reiki can be administered in almost any setting, those who receive Level One training can form informal support groups within the community to practice Reiki with each other.

> **REIKI AT MAYO CLINIC**
>
> Mayo Clinic introduced Reiki and healing touch — a similar therapeutic approach — into its practice over a decade ago, prompted by requests from patients who were interested in holistic therapies. You can read more about the pilot program on page 117. Mayo Clinic nurses offer these services through a volunteer program. Patients and their healthcare teams can make requests for either service, as inpatients or outpatients.

WHAT THE RESEARCH SHOWS

Reiki is used to treat a variety of conditions. However, it is challenging to study because comparing Reiki with a placebo is difficult. Still, one systematic review found Reiki was, in fact, better than placebo and has broad potential as a holistic practice. There's some evidence that Reiki helps with pain, fatigue and anxiety. And some research suggests that Reiki could have beneficial effects on blood pressure and heart rate.

Stress and anxiety
Several small studies found that Reiki reduced stress and anxiety, particularly in people preparing for medical procedures. The studies suggested that Reiki might be beneficial delivered in medical settings.

Pain and fatigue
One study found that Reiki helped reduce pain and fatigue in people undergoing dialysis. Another study found that Reiki, alone or in combination with acupressure, reduced the need for pain medications in people with cancer. Acupressure is similar to acupuncture, except that it applies pressure rather than needles to specific parts of the body.

Pain and anxiety
An in-depth review of several trials noted that Reiki effectively reduced pain and anxiety in adults but noted that larger studies are needed.

RISKS AND SAFETY CONCERNS
There are no significant risks involved in Reiki, but sometimes people have become emotional during a session. As they relax, they may think of certain things that lead to emotional release. "Sometimes Reiki can bring

up a wide array of emotions," says Abbey K. Metzger, also a nurse at Mayo Clinic who practices Reiki. "Reiki can be a way for people to open up, which may allow big emotions to surface. This shouldn't be interpreted as a negative experience, as sometimes those things need attending. This presents an opportunity to pause, reflect, and process."

More often, people just completely relax. It is not uncommon for people to achieve a state of deep rest, and even sleep, during a session.

OUR TAKE

Like healing touch, the benefits associated with Reiki may come from its ability to promote relaxation. Systematic scientific evidence of its efficacy is still lacking, but the experience of people who receive Reiki is typically positive. Learning Reiki also can enable a person to engage in self-healing or form a support group with others.

Rolfing

Rolfing, also referred to as Rolfing Structural Integration, SI or RSI, is a form of bodywork intended to alleviate discomfort and pain. It was developed more than 50 years ago by Ida Rolf, a chemist who had health problems and sought help in holistic practices.

Rolfing is based on the theory that the tissues surrounding your muscles become thickened and stiff as you get older. Aging also reduces the elasticity of your fascia — a thin layer of connective tissue that surrounds organs, blood vessels, bones, nerve fibers and muscles and holds them in place. This affects your posture and how well you're able to move.

Rolf recognized that the body isn't just a collection of separate parts but rather one unified system that is best treated as a whole. For example, the legs are aligned to the hips, the shoulders are aligned to the rib cage and the body is positioned over the feet. All of these joints and related tissues are connected to one another.

The primary concept behind Rolf's structural integration system is to help people achieve proper vertical alignment and efficient movement of these interconnected body parts. Her technique focuses on the fascia to release and realign the body, and to balance all of the body's components into a functioning coordinated whole.

To correct internal misalignments, Rolfing practitioners apply mild, direct pressure to the different parts of the body. They use slow, deep strokes to trigger the nervous system to reduce tension in related muscles and fascia. They may use their fingers, knuckles, thumbs, elbows and knees to slowly manipulate muscles and the tissues surrounding muscles and joints. This is meant to alter a person's posture and realign the body.

During a session, you typically lie on a treatment table, but you may be seated or standing. Your therapist may ask to you do specific movements as force is applied. This process is thought to restore flexibility, revitalize your energy and leave you feeling more comfortable, coordinated and agile.

In addition to improving posture and balance, Rolfing also may relieve stress and anxiety, and ease pain.

WHAT THE RESEARCH SAYS

One small study found that 10 Rolfing sessions were sufficient to significantly lessen neck pain and stiffness while also increasing range of motion. Another small study suggested that Rolfing could potentially be useful in reducing low back pain.

In addition to improving posture and balance, Rolfing also may relieve stress and anxiety, and ease pain.

Rolfing has been studied for the treatment of low back pain, cerebral palsy, impaired balance and chronic fatigue syndrome. But the available studies are small, and more reliable data are needed to show that it's an effective treatment for these conditions.

RISKS AND SAFETY CONCERNS

The deep friction massage traditionally performed with Rolfing techniques can be painful and even lead to bruising. However, newer techniques are gentler and less painful.

Because Rolfing involves manipulation of tissues deep beneath the skin, it should be avoided when any of the following are present:
- A bleeding disorder.
- Pregnancy.
- Broken bones.
- Osteoporosis.
- An implanted medical device such as a shunt or a pacemaker.
- Skin conditions that might be further irritated, such as eczema, psoriasis, infection, burns or open wounds.
- A blood clot deep in a leg vein, also known as deep vein thrombosis.

OUR TAKE

Some people find Rolfing to be useful in improving their posture or helping them to feel more agile. But the therapy also can be painful. If you have a specific underlying illness, such as advanced osteoporosis, the deep massage of Rolfing may pose some risk of harm.

If you're interested in Rolfing, talk to your healthcare team first. Mayo Clinic specialists typically don't use Rolfing to treat patients who are acutely ill, such as recovering from surgery or undergoing cancer treatments. But they do incorporate it as indicated in the outpatient setting.

Saunas

Sauna bathing, a tradition deeply rooted in Finnish culture, has been used for thousands of years for leisure, relaxation and wellness. But Finns are hardly the only ones to have embraced the benefits of sauna — other societies do too. Russians have *banyas*. Turks have *hammams*. Native Americans have sweat lodges. They have one thing in common: They all offer the opportunity to feel better through heat and sweat.

How do heat and sweat improve your well-being? There is, in fact, some science behind it.

During sauna use, people experience a short-term exposure to high temperatures, typically ranging from 113 to 212 degrees F. This causes some overheating, to which the body quickly mounts a protective cardiovascular, neuroendocrine and cellular response to maintain internal balance (homeostasis). Repeated sauna use teaches the body to adapt to heat and optimizes its response to future exposures, increasing the body's overall resilience. Moreover, due to the heat exposure in the sauna, the heart rate may increase up to 120 to 150 beats per minute, as much as it would during exercise. In that way, sauna use mimics physiological and protective responses induced by exercise.

HEALTH BENEFITS OF SAUNAS

In addition to temporarily lowering your blood pressure and promoting relaxation, sauna use may have positive antioxidant and anti-inflammatory effects on your heart, circulatory system and immune system.

Evidence suggests that frequent sauna bathing boosts cardiovascular fitness and protects against high blood pressure and systemic inflammation. It also may offer protection against neurodegenerative diseases. Recent research shows that regular sauna use may stave off dementia and Alzheimer's disease and foster healthy cognitive aging.

In addition, when you sweat, your body takes the opportunity to clear out toxins, including pesticides and heavy metals such as cadmium, lead and aluminum. If you feel refreshed and revitalized after a sauna visit, you indeed are. You just sweated out a load of substances you're better off without.

Sauna use also may boost production of endorphins, the body's feel-good chemicals, promoting feelings of relaxation and well-being and improving mental health.

Rejuvenate Spa at Mayo Clinic's Healthy Living Center features saunas as part of its other spa services, which include massage, facials, acupuncture, aromatherapy, hot tubs, yoga and body treatments. Learn more about Rejuvenate Spa at Mayo Clinic's Healthy Living Center: *https://healthyliving.mayoclinic.org/rejuvenate-spa.php*.

WHAT THE RESEARCH SAYS
Sauna use may offer tangible benefits for a wide range of conditions and symptoms.

Fibromyalgia
A 12-week thermal therapy that consisted of sauna use and underwater exercise in a warm treatment pool reduced pain in people with fibromyalgia.

Rheumatic conditions
Studies found that saunas, traditional and infrared ones, may ease pain and stiffness in people with rheumatic conditions such as arthritis and ankylosing spondylitis, all without harmful side effects.

Pneumonia
A recent study found that combining physical fitness with frequent visits to the sauna lowers risk of pneumonia, which may have implications for preventing respiratory-related illnesses such as COVID-19.

Common colds and asthma
Sauna bathing may improve breathing in people with asthma and chronic bronchitis, improving the overall function of the respiratory tract.

Stress reduction and disease prevention
A recent study found that saunas have a positive effect on people working in high-stress occupations, such as firefighters, police, military personnel and first responders. Chronic low-level stress causes inflammation and contributes to cardiac and metabolic health issues. The study noted sauna bathing as a potential countermeasure.

Healthy cognitive aging
One study found that men who used saunas 4 to 7 times a week had a 66% reduction in dementia compared to those who did it only once a week. A larger study confirmed this finding, noting that regular visits, such as 9 to 12 times a month, decreased dementia risk. A short stay (5 to 14 minutes) in temperatures between 175 and 194 degrees F was sufficient to make a difference. Another study noted the benefits of heat therapy for overall brain health and healthy cognitive aging.

INFRARED SAUNAS

If the heat of a traditional sauna is too much for you, you might consider an infrared sauna. A regular sauna uses heat to warm the air, which in turn warms your body. An infrared sauna uses infrared light to heat your body directly without warming the air around you.

Saunas trigger body reactions similar to those caused by moderate exercise, such as vigorous sweating and an increased heart rate. An infrared sauna gives these results at lower temperatures than a regular sauna.

No harmful effects have been reported with infrared saunas. So if you're thinking of trying a sauna to relax, an infrared sauna might be an option.

RISKS AND SAFETY CONCERNS

Although sauna bathing causes temporary physiological changes, it is generally well tolerated by most healthy adults and children.

Reasons to avoid saunas include unstable chest pain, a recent heart attack and severe aortic stenosis — a type of heart valve disease that reduces or blocks blood flow. Make sure to speak to your healthcare team before using a sauna if you have any of these conditions. Few heart attacks or sudden deaths occur in saunas. However, alcohol consumption during sauna bathing increases the risk of a dramatic drop in blood pressure, irregular heartbeat and sudden death, so don't drink alcohol in the sauna.

OUR TAKE

Overall, saunas are a helpful tool to promote holistic health and wellness, in addition to being a generally enjoyable experience. Regular sauna therapy — whether in the traditional radiant heat sauna or in an infrared unit — appears to be safe, and even mimics exercise to some extent.

Beyond pleasure and relaxation, sauna bathing has several health benefits, including reducing blood pressure, improving cardiovascular, respiratory and brain health, and alleviating pain in certain chronic conditions.

Use a sauna for an appropriate length of time to avoid overheating. If you have heart disease, consider discussing sauna use with your healthcare team first to ensure that it's a safe option for you.

Spinal manipulation

Spinal manipulation techniques have roots in practices going back a thousand years or more (see opposite page). According to some scholars, Greek physician Hippocrates was an early practitioner of spinal manipulation, using it "not only to reposition vertebrae, but also thereby to cure a wide variety of dysfunctions." In fact, the very word *chiropractic*, commonly used to describe spinal manipulation, comes from the Greek words *cheir*, meaning "hand," and *praktos*, meaning "done" — as in "done by hand."

Today, spinal manipulation often serves as a holistic alternative to surgical or drug interventions, typically for pain relief. Chiropractic treatment is widely recognized as one of the safest drug-free, noninvasive therapies available for decreasing back pain, neck pain, joint pain in the arms or legs and headaches. A similar holistic approach, osteopathic treatment, is used for conditions such as low back pain, migraines and carpal tunnel syndrome.

CHIROPRACTIC AND OSTEOPATHY: WHAT'S THE DIFFERENCE?

Chiropractic and osteopathy are two similar techniques for spinal manipulation, but there are a few differences.

Chiropractic

Chiropractic is a licensed healthcare profession that treats disorders by manual therapy, such as spinal manipulation. Chiropractic was founded in the late 1800s by Daniel David Palmer, a self-educated healer in the Mississippi River town of Davenport, Iowa. In 1897, he established the Palmer School of Chiropractic, which is still one of the most prominent chiropractic colleges in the nation.

Early chiropractic notions, such as Eastern views of qi, held that an innate vital force flows through the body's nervous system and that an impingement on that flow in the spinal column or elsewhere causes disease. Manipulating the spine essentially frees up that life force. Ultimately, however, Western chiropractic professions evolved with a greater musculoskeletal focus.

According to the American Chiropractic Association, today over 70,000 chiropractors are practicing in the United States, reportedly treating more than 35 million adults and children annually. According to past surveys, women are more likely than men to visit a chiropractor and

202   Mayo Clinic Guide to Holistic Health

HISTORY OF SPINAL MANIPULATION

Hippocrates, who is often referred to as the father of medicine, was the first physician to describe spinal manipulation techniques for the treatment of scoliosis. Galen, a Greek-born Roman physician, also used spinal manipulation to treat patients.

Avicenna, an ancient physician from Baghdad, included descriptions of Hippocrates' techniques in his medical text *The Book of Healing*. Later, these "bonesetting" techniques were passed down through generations within families, not only from father to son but also often from mother to daughter.

Spinal manipulation has been part of medicine in many world cultures, including in Asia and South America. It's also known to have been practiced by the Balinese of Indonesia, the Lomi-Lomi of Hawaii and the bonesetters of Nepal, Russia and Norway. It also made its way to the American Midwest, where in the second half of the 19th century it gave rise to two modern manipulation-based healing approaches, osteopathy and chiropractic.

people in the 45 to 64 age range are more likely than older or younger adults to seek chiropractic care.

Chiropractic is a highly regulated profession. Training requires classes in basic sciences, including anatomy and physiology, and supervised clinical experience in which students learn skills such as spinal assessment, adjustment techniques and making diagnoses.

To receive a doctor of chiropractic degree (D.C.), a person must complete 4 to 5 years at an accredited chiropractic college. Chiropractors also must pass a national board exam and any state tests before receiving a license to practice. Low back pain, neck pain and headaches are the most common problems for which people seek chiropractic adjustment.

Osteopathy

Osteopathy is a branch of medicine that treats disorders through manipulation and massage of the bones, joints and muscles. It was developed by Andrew Still, a self-trained bonesetter in the United States in the late 1800s. Still founded the American School of Osteopathy and established the *Journal of Osteopathy* in 1894.

As part of their modern education, doctors of osteopathy (D.O.) receive special training in the musculoskeletal system — the body's interconnected system of nerves, muscles and bones. Using osteopathy techniques, these professionals can effectively treat muscles and joints to relieve pain, promote healing and increase overall mobility.

Osteopathy is often used to treat muscle pain, but it also can help provide relief for patients with asthma, sinus disorders, carpal tunnel syndrome and migraines. In many cases, it can be used to complement, or even replace, drugs or surgery.

Early osteopathic concepts were similar to Eastern notions of qi, except that osteopaths believed the life force flowed through the vascular

EXPERT INSIGHT
A HOLISTIC ROUTINE

When the weary 30-something woman finally ended up in the office of chiropractor Ben Holmes, D.C., Ph.D., she was at the end of her rope. For the last eight months, she had been battling an odd pain for which nobody could identify a cause. Her pain affected her middle to lower back, but also her hip and lower abdomen. She had gone through a colonoscopy and an endoscopy. She had seen a liver specialist. She had seen a neurologist. She had tried physical therapy. None of that produced either a diagnosis or relief. The pain was affecting her family life and leaving her depressed. "It was a really dark time for her," says Dr. Holmes.

Spinal manipulation helped, but in addition Dr. Holmes recommended an array of holistic therapies specifically for the woman's needs. Besides spinal manipulation, her routine included yoga and myofascial release work — a type of massage that relaxes contracted muscles, improving blood flow and elasticity.

Once all three practices were combined into a holistic routine, the woman started feeling better. "It was very thrilling, enjoyable and meaningful to me, witnessing this change. And to think that I played a small part in this change," says Dr. Holmes. "I haven't seen her in 10 months, but I have been in contact with her, and she is doing great."

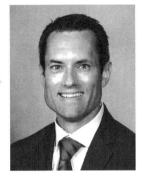

Ben Holmes, D.C., Ph.D.
Spine Center

system, alongside blood. That's why in the United States, osteopathy evolved into a profession similar to other fields of medicine, with few osteopaths focusing only on spinal manipulation. In Europe, however, the practice of osteopathy is more focused on spinal manipulation.

WHAT TO EXPECT DURING A CHIROPRACTOR VISIT
On your first visit, the chiropractor will likely take a detailed medical history from you, including the reasons for your visit. It's important to give your chiropractor a complete picture of your health, including whether you had an injury or surgery in the past, or if you have an implanted device such as a pacemaker. Your chiropractor will probably also examine your entire spine from neck to pelvis, and possibly other joints and parts of your body.

During a spinal manipulation, you lie down, either facedown, faceup or on your side. The chiropractor uses a controlled movement called a thrust manipulation to push a joint beyond its usual range of motion. You may hear popping or cracking sounds as your chiropractor moves your joints during the treatment session. The goal of the procedure is to improve spinal motion and improve your body's physical function.

Many chiropractors also use soft tissue manipulation techniques aimed to relax your muscles and joints to make manipulation easier and more pleasant. Some may use heated pads or ultrasonic equipment to aid relaxation. When spinal manipulation alone doesn't provide improvement or doesn't restore the full range of motion, chiropractors also may employ massage techniques to work on the muscles in the affected area.

Some chiropractors might recommend X-rays to see if there is any visible misalignment. Others go back to the original idea of unblocking the flow of a person's vital life force. They believe that the power of human touch is often better at detecting misalignment problems than

In a recent systematic review, researchers found that spinal manipulation is as effective as other common back-pain therapies, such as exercise and standard medical care.

imaging tests. Blockages won't appear on X-rays, but a good practitioner will likely sense them during the examination, proponents believe.

"At Mayo Clinic we use a technique called motion palpation," says Mayo Clinic chiropractor Ben Holmes, D.C., Ph.D. "The idea is that as we palpate the spine, we apply pressure to different parts of the spine and to different vertebrae to get a sense of where it moves. Does it move the way it's supposed to, and if not, how can I get it to move appropriately? We do that from the cervical spine all the way down to the sacrum and pelvis."

Chiropractors and osteopaths also may recommend specific exercises, lifestyle changes or other adjustments to treat your problem in a holistic way.

FINDING A QUALIFIED CHIROPRACTOR

Looking for a good chiropractor is similar to looking for a good doctor — you need to find one who understands your body, your challenges and your goals. Ask your healthcare team for a recommendation. Tap into your circle of family and friends. If possible, look for a chiropractor who works within a large healthcare system or a research institution.

When calling the chiropractor's office for the first time, ask how long an appointment usually lasts. It should not be very short, cautions Dr. Holmes. A promise of an in-and-out 10-minute visit should raise a red flag because it suggests the office is trying to recruit as many patients as possible. If the office is promising to cure all ailments, that's a red flag too. Generally, spinal manipulation is recommended for low back pain, neck pain and certain types of headaches.

The American Chiropractic Association maintains a database of professionals in different states at *https://handsdownbetter.org/find-a-doctor*. The American Osteopathic Association also offers a search function at *https://findado.osteopathic.org*. So does the American Academy of Osteopathy: *www.academyofosteopathy.org*.

WHAT THE RESEARCH SAYS

Studies show that spinal manipulation is an effective treatment for mild to moderate low back pain, neck pain and certain types of headaches. However, there's little evidence that spinal manipulation works for other conditions such as menstrual pain, sciatica or high blood pressure.

Back pain

Many high-quality studies have been conducted examining the effect of spinal manipulation on back pain. Most have found that it does help. In a recent systematic review, researchers studied 26 randomized controlled

Low back pain, neck pain and headaches are the most common problems for which people seek chiropractic adjustment.

trials that included more than 6,000 participants to determine what effect spinal manipulation has on chronic low back pain. In this review, researchers found that spinal manipulation is as effective as other common back-pain therapies, such as exercise and standard medical care. Another study found chiropractic care to be a cost-effective alternative to physical therapy.

Chronic back pain
A very recent study found that spinal manipulation can produce long-lasting pain relief in people with chronic low back pain.

Migraines
A systematic review and meta-analysis of investigations into spinal manipulation for migraine headache found that spinal manipulation reduced the number of days people experienced migraines.

RISKS AND SAFETY CONCERNS
Chiropractic adjustment is generally considered to be safe. It rarely causes discomfort and can be a holistic alternative to pharmaceutical and surgical interventions. However, it's not uncommon to feel sore for a day or two after treatment.

"The reason for that is the manipulation is restoring movement into different parts of the spine or parts of the body," says Dr. Holmes. Sometimes that movement is blocked by soft tissue or connective tissue resistance or tension, or even so-called adhesions, when tissues are "stuck together" that shouldn't be. As manipulation breaks these blocks and adhesions it causes a bit of injury, akin to what you may experience with exercise. "We consider it a good injury because it leads to healing and improved mobility, but it can cause an inflammatory response and pain," Dr. Holmes says. "So we recommend patients apply ice to the area that was manipulated, and that can help limit the inflammatory response. Often, when I'm finished with my session, I let my patients rest for about five minutes with ice on areas that I manipulated."

Serious complications associated with chiropractic adjustment are rare but may include a herniated disk or compression of the nerves in your lower spinal column. In very rare instances, neck manipulation may cause a type of stroke known as vertebral artery dissection, caused by a blockage in the vertebral arteries. Vertebral arteries are located on both sides of the spine. Such strokes are extremely rare, at the rate of 1 in 1 million cases. It is also not known whether the manipulation actually causes the stroke because patients may have prior arterial plaques that could block blood flow s.

Sometimes spinal manipulation isn't recommended, as it may cause more harm than good. Don't seek chiropractic adjustment if you have any of the following:
- Severe osteoporosis.
- Numbness, tingling, or loss of strength in an arm or leg.
- Cancer in your spine.
- An increased risk of stroke.
- A known bone abnormality in the upper neck.

OUR TAKE
When performed by someone who's trained and licensed to deliver that type of care, spinal manipulation is safe and effective. When used appropriately, the most common side effect is local discomfort, which is generally short-lived. Overall, spinal manipulation is a relatively safe option that has shown benefits for musculoskeletal conditions. Low back pain, neck pain and headaches are the most common problems for which people seek chiropractic adjustment. Spinal manipulation is also reasonable in terms of cost, as it is typically covered by insurance.

However, not everyone responds to chiropractic adjustments. Much depends on your particular situation. If your symptoms don't begin to improve after several weeks of treatments, chiropractic adjustment might not be the best option for you.

Tai chi

You may have heard of tai chi as a martial art. It did indeed originate in China as a self-defense system that evolved from the ancient practice of qigong (see page 186) — a way to harness qi (CHEE), the life energy that, according to traditional Chinese medicine, flows through the channels inside the human body, nourishing organs and tissues. Tai chi is a type of qigong, but qigong is not a type of tai chi.

Today, tai chi is commonly performed as an exercise for health promotion and rehabilitation. It typically involves integrated physical postures, focused attention and controlled breathing. Modern tai chi looks like a series of slowly performed, dance-like postures that flow into one another. Tai chi (the phrase translates as "grand ultimate") encompasses concentration, balance, muscle relaxation and relaxed breathing.

Tai chi is popular in the United States. From 2007 to 2017, tai chi and qigong practice among U.S. adults grew by more than 60%. The practice is popular among people who appreciate a useful, easy and cost-effective way to exercise.

HOW TO FIND A QUALIFIED INSTRUCTOR

Tai chi instructors don't need a license and there's no national standard for tai chi certification. However, various tai chi organizations offer training and certification programs, with differing criteria and certification levels. If you're considering taking a tai chi class or joining a group, ask the teacher what type of certification they have and what type of tai chi they practice. Also, let them know your health status and goals for the class. That way, you can see if you are a good fit.

FIVE STYLES

There are five common styles of tai chi:
- Chen
- Yang
- Wu
- Hao
- Sun

The most-taught form of tai chi is Yang, due to its slow and gentle movement and pace.

TAI CHI | Therapies A–Z **209**

For tai chi beginners, the focus is almost always on correcting posture, calming the mind and using the breath to guide the movements. Typically, the movements are graceful, circular and within the natural range of motion.

A tai chi session may be as short as a few minutes or as much as half an hour or even longer. As with qigong (see page 186), it's believed that the best time to practice is in the morning as the sun rises. This is when the yang energy is active, which helps jump-start the day. Alternatively, you may choose to practice calming movements in the evening, to unwind from the day.

WHAT THE RESEARCH SHOWS
Evidence supporting the physical and mental health benefits of tai chi is growing. Research finds that it can improve balance in older adults and people with Parkinson's disease, as well as reduce pain from fibromyalgia, arthritis and cancer. It may ease breathing in people with chronic obstructive pulmonary disease and aid in rehabilitation from COVID-19. It also may uplift mood and ease depression.

Physical fitness
One study found that when older adults practiced tai chi for 12 weeks, their well-being, physical fitness and self-control improved significantly compared to the group that didn't engage in the exercise.

Balance
One study concluded that tai chi can improve balance in older adults and prevent them from falling. Moreover, feeling stronger made them more self-confident and less afraid of falling.

Strength
A research effort that followed 167 community-dwelling adults who engaged in tai chi twice a week for 12 weeks found that they grew stronger and less frail.

Parkinson's disease
Evidence suggests that tai chi can help people with Parkinson's disease maintain their sense of balance. Falls are common events in people with Parkinson's and are a major concern. One systematic review found that practicing tai chi may help decrease the number of falls in people with Parkinson's.

Chronic obstructive pulmonary disease (COPD)
COPD causes permanent damage to the lungs, blocking the airflow and

resulting in breathing problems. One study found that combining conventional lung rehabilitation techniques with tai chi lessened inflammation and other symptoms and resulted in better breathing and greater exercise ability.

COVID-19
Another study found tai chi to be an effective way to cope with COVID-19 during the pandemic. Tai chi is believed to have beneficial effects on inflammation, immunity and the respiratory system.

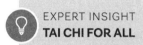

EXPERT INSIGHT
TAI CHI FOR ALL

Alexander Do, L.Ac., an acupuncturist at Mayo Clinic, has been practicing tai chi for over 20 years. While many think of tai chi as a self-defense practice, it is a system of exercise that nearly anyone can do.

The best thing about tai chi is that it can be started at any age. The exercises follow the principles of the life energy qi and the two opposing forces of yin and yang. When yin and yang are balanced, qi can be cultivated and flow freely.

Tai chi incorporates a wide range of physical movements that are coordinated, slow, meditative, flowing and in sync with the mind and breath. Tai chi is practiced with the intention to strengthen and relax the body and mind. "These practices are ideal for health and healing, as the goal is to harmonize our bodies internally and externally," Do says.

Beginner tai chi exercises are quite simple, Do says. For example, imagine you are putting a light blanket on your bed. Slowly bring your arms up with palms relaxed and your fingers pointing downward as you move. Then as your wrists and elbows drop down naturally, slowly bring your arms down.

"So you basically create a wave as your wrists and elbows go up, and then when they go down," Do says. You do it slowly and you breathe in sync with your movements. "When you slow your body down, your heart rate will slow down and your cortisol, the stress hormone, will drop," Do explains. "Your body and your brain will start promoting the relaxation response." The main purpose of tai chi and the similar practice of qigong is to make a conscious effort to control your body instead of your body controlling you.

Depression and mood
Several studies noted tai chi's beneficial effect on thinking and memory, also called cognition, and mood. One research effort analyzed 12 trials with a total of 731 participants to assess whether tai chi can help ease depression. It concluded that the practice can be a valid alternative therapy for reducing depression in middle-aged and older adults. Another study found that practicing tai chi had an overall positive effect on cognition and physical functioning.

Cancer-related symptoms
A number of studies suggest that tai chi may be helpful in decreasing cancer fatigue, lowering blood pressure and normalizing blood sugar in diabetes. But the studies were small and not well designed, so more research is needed.

RISKS AND SAFETY CONCERNS
Tai chi appears to be safe. A 2019 review of 24 studies and close to 2,000 participants found that practicing tai chi did not produce any harmful effects, save for minor aches and pains.

There are no published studies on the safety of tai chi during pregnancy, but light physical activities are usually desirable during pregnancy, as long as appropriate precautions are taken. Tai chi may help with blood circulation, balance, coordination, strength, relaxation and mental health during pregnancy. More research in these areas is needed. If you are pregnant, talk with your healthcare team before starting tai chi.

OUR TAKE
Growing evidence supports the conclusion that tai chi can provide many physical and mental health benefits. It can improve balance and reduce the number of falls in older adults and people with Parkinson's disease. It may improve mood and reduce depression and fatigue. It may ease breathing for people with chronic obstructive pulmonary disease and aid in rehabilitation from COVID-19. Cost is usually the price of a class. But you also can use an app or videos on YouTube to learn tai chi. You can practice alone or with a group of friends. Tai chi can be a convenient and inexpensive way to restore wellness and promote health.

Tui na / Chinese massage

Tui na (the phrase means "pushing and pulling" in Chinese) is one of the oldest-known healing systems and is a form of massage. It has been used in China for thousands of years. It consists of a series of maneuvers that include pressing, kneading and grasping, and range from light stroking to deep tissue work. Practitioners also incorporate elements of acupressure — a technique similar to acupuncture that applies pressure rather than needles to specific parts of the body — as part of the treatment strategy.

TUI NA IN CHINA

These early massage techniques evolved to help people who experienced physically challenging lives, were exposed to the elements and were prone to frequent injuries. People discovered that manipulating skin and tissue could have beneficial effects. Pressing could stop bleeding, and rubbing could ease pain and reduce swelling, so they adapted these practices into their lives.

In China, there are many types of *tui na*, each with its own style, strength and therapeutic effects. These styles developed from the health needs of residents and were passed down through generations. As the practice has spread to the West, training in and the practice of *tui na* are continuing to develop and evolve to suit the health needs of local people.

Therapists who practice *tui na* today go through extensive training, learning to perform very specific movements. Therapists practice the movements repeatedly, usually on bags of rice, before they begin working with people.

HOW IT WORKS

Tui na uses the meridian system, a network of 14 energy channels or pathways in the human body. Through these channels flows the vital energy or

Early tui na techniques evolved to help people who experienced physically challenging lives.

life force called qi (CHEE), discussed on page 65. Proper flow of qi balances and regulates your spiritual, emotional, mental and physical health. A blockage of qi prevents it from nourishing organs. Removing blocks by stimulating acupoints on the meridians restores its flow.

The goal of *tui na* is to reestablish the normal flow of qi through the application of massage and manipulation techniques at the acupressure points. *Tui na* is commonly used together with acupuncture, or instead of acupuncture when people are uncomfortable using needles.

Tui na is often applied to limited areas of the body. Unlike most forms of massage, Chinese massage generally isn't a light, relaxing experience. The techniques can be quite forceful and intense, and even a bit painful. At Mayo Clinic some acupuncturists practice *tui na*, usually performing only a few quick maneuvers along with needle placement.

WHAT THE RESEARCH SAYS

Tui na is often used to treat injuries; joint, muscle and other orthopedic problems; and chronic pain. But it's also used for some internal disorders.

AI-ASSISTED *TUI NA*

Meet EMMA, a massage provider that also happens to be a robot. EMMA stands for Expert Manipulative Massage Automation. Developed by AiTreat, a startup in Singapore, EMMA's robotic arms are designed to give people therapeutic *tui na*. Mayo Clinic is conducting clinical evaluations of EMMA.

EMMA's artificial intelligence system uses sensors to measure muscle stiffness and calculate the acupoints in each person's body. It also uses data points from many different body types and sizes to offer a customized therapeutic strategy. Its arms, also called modules, have a soft-touch surface that's warmed to between 100.4 and 104 degrees F to mimic human touch.

Robotic massage can help *tui na* therapists by performing some of the manual efforts involved in this type of massage. "We want the therapist to do the assessment and the positioning, but then the robot can take over some of the repetitive work," says Brent A. Bauer, M.D., director of research for the Mayo Clinic Integrative Medicine and Health program. Watch a video of EMMA at work on YouTube: *www.youtube.com/watch?v=GXEXUCCCGzI&t=7s*.

Of the limited research that has been done on *tui na*, studies suggest it may be effective in helping treat several conditions.

High blood pressure
Some evidence indicates that, when used with medications, *tui na* may help lower blood pressure in people who have high blood pressure. However, researchers are cautious about these findings because of the poor quality of information available.

Low back pain
A randomized controlled trial showed that *tui na* combined with herbal ointment helped treat low back pain more effectively than massage therapy on its own. These researchers were also cautious about the results, echoing the need for longer-term, better-quality studies. Mayo Clinic scientists are working with research teams in Singapore and China to study the use of *tui na* for low back pain.

Dyspepsia
A review of randomized controlled trials involving over 1,000 participants looked at *tui na* therapy for dyspepsia, more commonly referred to as indigestion. The review showed that *tui na* helped decrease overall symptoms of dyspepsia.

Musculoskeletal and joint conditions
One small study found that *tui na* reduced pain and possibly increased muscle strength in people with knee osteoarthritis.

A more recent study found that *tui na* lessened pain and muscle stiffness in athletes, while increasing joint range of motion and performance. The study also noted that *tui na* helped dampen inflammation caused by sports injuries.

Other evidence suggests that *tui na* can be effective in treating temporomandibular joint (TMJ) disorder, which causes pain and dysfunction in the jaw joint and the muscles that control jaw movement.

OUR TAKE
Tui na has been part of a comprehensive traditional Chinese medicine system for thousands of years. Clinical studies also supply some evidence of its positive effects on health and wellness. More research is needed to understand *tui na*'s full benefits. In the meantime, it may provide care to people who aren't getting full relief from conventional treatment.

Virtual reality

Wouldn't it be great to don a pair of rose-colored glasses and instantly whisk away your stress and worry? Unfortunately, there are no gadgets that can do that. But the good news is that modern technology is starting to approach that level of "magic." You can't don a pair of fairy-tale glasses, but you can put on a virtual reality (VR) headset, which can mess with your head — in a good way.

This form of immersive experience allows you to place yourself in situations that mimic what happens in real life. When you wear a VR headset, you experience certain environments, actions or interactions as if they were happening in a three-dimensional world. VR headsets have grown in popularity in recent years, so you may have already experienced them at events, museums or special exhibits.

Besides offering entertainment, virtual reality settings can serve as a form of therapy, especially for certain conditions such as anxiety, PTSD or various phobias, as well as for stress and pain relief.

VIRTUAL REALITY EXPOSURE THERAPY

Virtual reality exposure therapy (VRET) is a specialized treatment that can mimic various real-life stressors but poses no real harm. It's like a high-tech version of exposure therapy, which is commonly used to treat anxiety disorders and obsessive-compulsive disorder. The idea is to teach you how to approach feared and avoided situations in a gradual, predictable, controllable and repetitive manner.

It works by exposing people to situations, thoughts, or memories that provoke anxiety or fear — but in safe settings where the participant can take the headset off at any moment. VRET is particularly advantageous for situations that are hard to re-create in real life, such as combat conditions for veterans or plane turbulence for those with flight phobias.

WHAT THE RESEARCH SHOWS

Research into various forms of virtual reality therapy has exploded in the recent past, in large part because the technology has become more accessible and affordable.

Scientists have found that VRET can be useful for PTSD, certain phobias and performance anxiety. Virtual reality also may be useful for stress relief and pain management.

PTSD and certain phobias
Evidence suggests that VRET can reduce PTSD symptoms, in some cases significantly. Some studies also found that the positive effects of VRET therapy can last a long time — for example, six months to a year. A growing body of research finds that VRET can be an effective treatment for various forms of anxiety, including social anxiety and anxiety during airplane flights. It also can be used to treat phobias, such as fear of spiders.

Stress relief
Some studies suggest that immersion in 3D virtual reality, such as in nature scenes, or in mixed reality, where participants interact with virtual animals, may help relieve stress. Young adults who participated in studies of virtual reality found that it did help relieve stress and was also time-effective.

During the COVID-19 pandemic, Mayo Clinic investigated whether VR immersion therapy with guided nature-based imagery in the middle of the working day could help healthcare professionals cope with heightened stress. The study, though small, found that a 10-minute virtual "walk through the woods" reduced nervousness and anxiety, and enhanced calmness and focus.

Pain relief
Medical scientists are also investigating the use of virtual reality to relieve pain. Study results are mixed so far, indicating the need for more research. But there is evidence that virtual reality can help relieve acute pain in a hospital setting and also may help with chronic pain management. Another area where immersive virtual reality may be therapeutic is helping children and adolescents cope with the pain of cancer and its treatment.

RISKS AND SAFETY CONCERNS
Overall, virtual reality seems to be safe, but it may not be for everybody. Some people may experience so-called simulator sickness, also known as cyber sickness. The symptoms are similar to those of motion-induced sickness, such as nausea or drowsiness, but tend to be less severe.

OUR TAKE
Virtual reality is emerging as a potentially effective treatment for specific conditions such as anxiety, stress and pain. It appears to have few major side effects, but more research is needed. As it becomes more accessible and affordable, it may become a holistic alternative to medications or a complementary therapy to more traditional medical interventions.

Yoga

Although it first began as a spiritual practice in India many thousands of years ago, yoga has become popular as a way of promoting physical and mental well-being. It is a mind-body practice that offers many holistic benefits. Recently, when someone in the yoga world posed the question "Is yoga a therapy or a lifestyle?" the answer from an expert was: "Yoga is therapy for lifestyles!"

A 2017 national survey found that 1 in 7 American adults practiced yoga in the past 12 months. Among children age 4 to 17, it was about 1 in 12. The type of yoga practiced in the United States typically emphasizes physical postures, called asanas; breathing techniques, called pranayama; and meditation, called dhyana. Overall, yoga is viewed as an exercise not only for the physical body but also for the mind and spirit. It has become a popular way of promoting physical and mental well-being. There are many different yoga styles, ranging from gentle practices to physically demanding ones.

Yoga and two practices of Chinese origin — qigong and tai chi — are sometimes called meditative movement practices. All three practices include both meditative elements and physical ones. Read more about qigong and tai chi on pages 186-189 and 209-212.

BENEFITS OF YOGA

Depression, anxiety, stress and insomnia are among the most common reasons people turn to holistic practices such as yoga. Yoga helps you relax, slow your breath and focus on the present. These actions help lower blood pressure, cortisol levels, breathing rate and heart rate, and they can increase blood flow to the intestines and vital organs.

Yoga aims to achieve a calm mind, create a sense of well-being, improve self-confidence and attentiveness, and foster an optimistic outlook on life.

Yoga can provide three primary benefits that a typical gym routine may not provide: improved nervous system function, improved joint range of motion and improved dynamic balance.

Improved nervous system function

Since yoga is based on breathing, parts of the nervous system are affected when you control your breathing and lengthen your exhalations. This is cued throughout particular yoga sequences. Specifically, yoga can help

218 Mayo Clinic Guide to Holistic Health

lower the fight-or-flight (sympathetic) response and improve the body's rest-and-digest (parasympathetic) response.

Practicing slow, controlled breathing stimulates the body's vagus nerve, which takes information about your current state of relaxation and relays it to the rest of the body, including the brain. One area affected when the vagus nerve is stimulated is the parasympathetic nervous system, which controls the body's rest-and-digestion functions. The mindful breathing practiced in yoga increases the activity of the parasympathetic system. As a result, yoga lowers the heart rate, improves digestion and quality of sleep, and strengthens the immune system. Another benefit is reduced stress.

Improved joint range of motion
The difference between flexibility and active range of motion is important. Think of flexibility as how much a muscle can be passively stretched. In contrast, range of motion is the extent to which muscles can be used to control a joint's movement.

It's not uncommon these days for people to report neck and back pain and poor range of motion in their middle (thoracic) spine due to constant sitting, typing on computers and looking down at cellphones. Yoga is excellent for improving thoracic range of motion because many poses involve extending the body through the rib cage and using strength to hold these postures.

Yoga incorporates all four motions of the spine: flexion, extension, rotation and side-bending. Therefore, yoga can help prevent stiffness and disuse that can occur with age. Being able to control the available range of motion in joints is crucial to good posture and decreasing the risk of injury.

Improved dynamic balance
Think of balance like a muscle. It can be improved with different exercises, similar to improving your muscular strength by lifting weights.

Keep in mind that every person has a different body with different abilities, so you may need to modify yoga postures to match your capabilities.

Balance is a complex system, requiring three parts: the sensation of the foot on the ground, or proprioception; vision; and the inner ear, or vestibular system. These three parts tell the brain where the head is in space, and they work together to control both static and dynamic balance.

Yoga trains the proprioception and visual systems to improve balance. Depending on the pose, cues are sent to focus, for instance, on the foot rooted to the ground. When you concentrate in an attempt to maintain contact, the big toe, little toe and heel form a tripod of sorts, which in turn helps focus the proprioception portion of balance.

In yoga, you may hear the term *drishti*, which refers to obtaining a focused gaze or focus point in the mind. The concept comes into play as people aim to hold a pose with their eyes closed. Certain poses become more challenging with eyes closed, which improves the visual part of balance.

Also, moving back and forth between poses without fully touching a limb to the ground can increase the ability to dynamically move and not lose balance. Over time, this will often reduce the risk of falling while walking on uneven ground or turning quickly.

LEARNING YOGA

Although you can learn yoga from books and videos, beginners usually find it helpful to learn with an instructor. Classes also offer camaraderie and friendship, which are important to overall well-being.

Keep in mind that every person has a different body with different abilities, so you may need to modify yoga postures to match your capabilities. That's another reason to work with an instructor, who can offer modifications to prevent sprains and strains that may occur if you push your limits too much. Choosing an instructor who is experienced and who understands your needs is important to practice yoga safely and

 Yoga seems to help alleviate chronic conditions, such as depression, pain, anxiety and insomnia, and reduce risk for chronic diseases, such as heart disease and high blood pressure.

effectively. A qualified instructors will understand and encourage you to explore but not exceed your personal limits.

When you find a class that sounds interesting, talk with the instructor so you know what to expect. Questions to ask include:

- What are the instructor's qualifications? Where did they train and how long have they been teaching?
- Does the instructor have experience working with students with your needs or health concerns? If you have a sore knee or an aching shoulder, can the instructor help you find poses that won't aggravate your condition?
- How demanding is the class? Is it suitable for beginners? Will it be easy enough to follow along if it's your first time?
- What can you expect from the class? Is it aimed at your needs, such as stress management or relaxation, or is it geared toward something else?

WHAT THE RESEARCH SAYS

Evaluating research on the health effects of yoga can be challenging because differences in the types of yoga used in research studies may affect study results. So far, a number of studies have shown that yoga may help reduce stress and anxiety. It also can enhance your mood and overall sense of well-being. Practicing yoga may improve balance, flexibility, range of motion and strength. Yoga also seems to help alleviate chronic conditions, such as depression, pain, anxiety and insomnia, and reduce risk for chronic diseases, such as heart disease and high blood pressure.

Headaches

A systematic review evaluated yoga's effectiveness for headaches. Overall, the investigators found evidence that yoga can reduce headache frequency, duration and pain intensity, but not in all headache types. Patients with tension-type headaches reported significant benefits, but migraine patients did not.

Overall wellness

One study found that yogic practices enhance muscular strength and body flexibility, and they promote and improve respiratory and cardiovascular function. Additionally, the study found that yoga helped reduce stress, anxiety, depression and chronic pain. It also improved people's sleep patterns and enhanced their overall well-being and quality of life.

Immune system health
A recent large-scale genomic study found that people who took part in a meditation retreat where they practiced yoga had a dramatic boost in their immune system performance. They demonstrated an increased activity in genes related to a molecule called interferon, which helps cells fight off viruses. Notably, this enhancement occurred without activating the inflammatory part of the immune system.

Cancer
A number of studies and comprehensive literature reviews found yoga to be a beneficial intervention for people with breast cancer and other types of cancer. Practicing yoga appears to reduce fatigue, nausea, vomiting, anxiety, depression and distress while improving sleep and overall quality of life.

Irritable bowel syndrome
Several studies investigated the effects of yoga on people with irritable bowel syndrome (IBS), a chronic debilitating condition that can severely affect the quality of life. One study found yoga to have beneficial physical and mental effects. Another study found that yoga delivered via telehealth during the COVID-19 pandemic improved IBS symptoms and quality of life.

Blood pressure
A review by Mayo Clinic researchers found that yoga practiced a few times a week can be an effective lifestyle therapy for reducing blood pressure. The study also noted that greatest blood pressure reduction benefits were gained when breathing techniques, meditation and mental relaxation were combined.

RISKS AND SAFETY CONCERNS
Mayo Clinic also conducted an investigation of yoga risks. Some yoga poses — such as headstand, shoulder stand, lotus and half lotus (seated cross-legged positions), forward bend, backward bend and handstand — can be physically demanding. They may not be achievable by everyone. Some of them can cause injuries, including spine injuries.

Other common yoga mishaps include sprains and strains. The parts of the body most commonly injured are the knee or lower leg. However, many yoga injuries are due to repetitive strain and therefore may be preventable. Older adults may need to be particularly cautious when practicing yoga. The rate of yoga-related injuries treated in emergency departments is higher in people age 65 and older than in younger adults.

Yoga helps improve balance, posture, muscle strength, attention and mood. However, certain health conditions may require more caution while practicing yoga.

To reduce your chances of getting hurt while doing yoga:
- Practice yoga under the guidance of a qualified instructor. Learning yoga on your own without supervision has been associated with increased risks.
- If you're new to yoga, avoid advanced practices such as headstands, shoulder stands, the lotus position and forceful breathing.
- Be aware that hot yoga has special risks related to overheating and dehydration.
- Pregnant women, older adults and people with health conditions should talk with their healthcare providers and the yoga instructor about their individual needs. They may need to avoid or modify some yoga poses and practices. Some of the health conditions that may call for modifications in yoga include preexisting injuries, such as knee or hip injuries, lumbar spine disease, severe high blood pressure, balance issues and glaucoma.

Proceed with caution if you have any of the following conditions:
- A herniated disk.
- Eye conditions, including glaucoma.
- Pregnancy (yoga is generally considered safe during pregnancy, but some poses may need to be avoided).
- Severe balance problems.
- Severe osteoporosis.
- Uncontrolled high blood pressure.

OUR TAKE

Yoga is generally considered a safe form of physical activity for healthy people when performed properly, under the guidance of a qualified instructor. It helps improve balance, posture, muscle strength, attention and mood. However, certain health conditions may require that you use more caution while practicing yoga or abstain from the more demanding exercises. If you have concerns about starting yoga, discuss them with your healthcare team.

PART 3

Tool kit

We hope you have found this book to be thought-provoking and informative. We also hope that you've been challenged to take some positive steps toward improving your health.

As you're able, try to incorporate what you've learned so far into your daily routine. The therapies discussed in this book, from paying more attention to your diet to adding massage to your weekly schedule, can play a critical role in your personal health — mind, body and spirit.

At the same time, trying to adopt a healthier lifestyle can seem a bit daunting. One of the many questions you may have is how to begin. This last part of the book offers you a tool kit to get you started. You'll learn how to:

- Assess your current health and health goals.
- Take concrete steps toward more holistic health.
- Practice holistic health on any budget.
- Draft your healthcare team.
- Examine and apply available research.

ASSESS YOUR HEALTH AND SET YOUR GOALS

Whether you're ready to forge ahead or are still a little unsure of next steps, it helps to pull back for a moment to get a bird's-eye view of the path forward. Stop and think: What do you want your healthy life to look like? Once you have that picture in mind, the possibilities you see are your goals. Then think about ways you can achieve your goals based on what you've learned in this book.

To get you started, try answering the questions on the next few pages. They can help you assess your current health and think through what's important to you. They can also help you consider your whole-health fundamentals, the types of holistic medicine you'd like to try, why you would like to try them and what you hope to accomplish in adding holistic therapies to your overall wellness plan.

Many healthcare institutions use a form similar to this for patients who are visiting an integrative medicine department for the first time. You can make a copy of your answers and take it to your next appointment with your healthcare team to get your conversation about holistic care and integrative medicine started.

GENERAL HEALTH

On average, how would you describe your overall health?
☐ Excellent ☐ Very good ☐ Good ☐ Fair ☐ Poor

On average, how would you describe your diet?
☐ Excellent ☐ Very good ☐ Good ☐ Fair ☐ Poor

On average, what is your usual level of physical activity?
☐ Almost no activity (mainly sitting)
☐ Mild activity (walking short periods, not lifting or carrying)
☐ Moderate activity (walking a lot, not lifting or carrying)
☐ Heavy activity (running, lifting or carrying)

How many days a week do you get at least 30 minutes of brisk activity?
☐ 0-2 days
☐ 3-4 days
☐ 5-7 days

On average, how would you describe your sleep?
☐ Excellent ☐ Very good ☐ Good ☐ Fair ☐ Poor

Do you wake up feeling refreshed?
☐ Yes ☐ No

Do you fall asleep easily during the day?
☐ Yes ☐ No

Has anyone told you that you snore or hold your breath during the night?
☐ Yes ☐ No

How would you rate your energy level?
☐ Very low ☐ Low ☐ Moderate ☐ High ☐ Very high

What are your main concerns in terms of your health? Select up to four topics that are on your mind.

☐ Disease prevention ☐ Sleep problems
☐ Pain ☐ Cancer
☐ Fatigue ☐ Heart disease
☐ Stress ☐ Other(s) _____
☐ Anxiety ☐ Other(s) _____
☐ Fibromyalgia ☐ Other(s) _____

EMOTIONAL WELL-BEING

How would you rate your stress level?
- ☐ Very low
- ☐ Low
- ☐ Moderate
- ☐ High/nearly constant
- ☐ Very high/all the time

How would you rate your anxiety level?

☐ Very low ☐ Low ☐ Moderate ☐ High ☐ Very high

What are the biggest stressors in your life?

_____

_____

_____

What steps do you take to cope with stress?

_____

_____

_____

How often do you practice a relaxation program?
- ☐ Not at all
- ☐ A few times a month
- ☐ A few times a week
- ☐ Most days of the week
- ☐ Every day

Which relaxation programs do you practice? (Mark all that apply.)

☐ Prayer	☐ Music
☐ Meditation	☐ Art
☐ Yoga	☐ Reading
☐ Guided imagery	☐ Other(s) _____
☐ Deep breathing	☐ Other(s) _____

228   Mayo Clinic Guide to Holistic Health

CONNECTION WITH NATURE

How often do you get outside for more than a few minutes?
☐ Not at all
☐ A few times a month
☐ A few times a week
☐ Most days of the week
☐ Every day

How often do you see plants and animals?
☐ Not at all
☐ A few times a month
☐ A few times a week
☐ Most days of the week
☐ Every day

MEANING AND PURPOSE

What brings you joy and meaning in your life?

_____

_____

_____

_____

On average, how would you describe your spiritual well-being?
☐ Excellent   ☐ Very good   ☐ Good   ☐ Fair   ☐ Poor

On average, how would you describe your relationships?
☐ Excellent   ☐ Very good   ☐ Good   ☐ Fair   ☐ Poor

On average, how would you describe your work-life balance?
☐ Excellent   ☐ Very good   ☐ Good   ☐ Fair   ☐ Poor

HEALTH GOALS

What are some goals you have for your health?

For example, "I want to feel less stress," "I want to sleep better," or "I want to enjoy my relationships more." Often these goals are related, but note a specific one that you'd like to work on first. You might be surprised at how working on one aspect of your health can positively impact other aspects.

What are some whole-health fundamentals you can adopt or improve to help you reach your goal?

For example, if you want to minimize stress, you might opt for going to bed at a set time so you get enough sleep. Or you might want to take regular opportunities to commune with nature, even if it means just sticking your nose out the window to sniff the air.

What holistic therapies do you already use or have you tried?

(Examples include supplements, meditation, acupuncture, massage.)

Which therapies would you like to try?

_____

_____

_____

_____

What are some easy ways to incorporate one or two of these therapies into your regular schedule?

_____

_____

_____

_____

5 STEPS FOR MOVING FORWARD

Once you've assessed where you're at and where you would like to be, take these steps.

Make a commitment

Often, people find that writing down goals can help them make — and keep — healthy habits. Because life can get hectic and personal wellness may end up at the bottom of your list of priorities, you may find it helpful to record your commitment to health and quality of life where you can see it every day. Add wellness activities to your calendar just as you would any other important meeting or event. When they show up on your smartphone or computer, don't dismiss them. Learn how to prioritize your wellness commitments so that other activities don't intrude on them or keep you from following through.

Start small

Choose one or two therapies from this book that resonate with you or that target an area of concern. For example, if you have fibromyalgia, adding a weekly massage to your wellness regimen may be a good first step.

Keep in mind that if you start off trying to do too much at one time, you might get overwhelmed and discouraged. Instead, start small. For example, add 20 minutes of tai chi to your morning routine a few days a week, or 10 minutes of meditation each night before you go to bed. Make it an appointment like you do anything else that's important to remember.

Stick with it

None of the approaches in this book will create significant changes in your health overnight. In some cases, it may take several weeks before you begin to see benefits. Try to give any new therapy at least four to six weeks to pay off.

Reassess

Once you've made a change, ask yourself if the change is helping you as much as you'd hoped it would. If the answer is yes, keep going! If you're not seeing the improvements you'd hoped to see, don't despair. Talk with your healthcare team or instructor to see if there are things you can do that might yield better results. If you still don't see benefits, it may be time to try something else. Keep exploring until you find practices that fit you and your needs.

Grow

Nurture all aspects of your life — mind, body and spirit. If you started out small, you stuck with it and you're finding that a certain integrative

232 Mayo Clinic Guide to Holistic Health

> How you view the world around you
> and the everyday events in your life
> can make a significant difference
> in your overall well-being.

therapy is helping you, it may be time to expand. Consider selecting another area of your personal wellness that might benefit from greater attention, and follow the same steps — make a commitment, start small, stick with it and then reassess.

At the same time, realize that people are generally drawn to something new. If what you have been doing for a period of time doesn't have the same spark for you that it once did, trying something new may be just what you need to reinvigorate your wellness routine.

Ideally, this book has illustrated why therapies such as massage, meditation and acupuncture are valuable. Now it's up to you to find out what meets your individual needs and fits your personal lifestyle.

One more note: Make your journey into holistic health a team effort. Talk with your healthcare team about what you've learned. From there, work together to make sure any changes you're contemplating won't interfere with the good care you're already receiving.

HOLISTIC HEALTH ON A BUDGET

Affordability is a significant issue for many people when it comes to healthcare. Understandably, you may question if holistic health and integrative therapies can fit into your lifestyle from a cost perspective.

While it's true that some integrative therapies, such as massage and acupuncture, do involve cost, many do not. Here is a list of integrative medicine techniques that cost little or nothing that you can do on your own.

Art therapy

Whether you're drawing, painting, sculpting or producing art in another form, creating art or even interpreting artwork can be therapeutic. With art therapy, you can spend as little or as much money as you like to find the medium that works best for you. Learn more about art therapy on page 86.

Tool kit **233**

Deep breathing

Breathing is something you do naturally without giving it much thought. But by breathing through your diaphragm, slowly and deeply, you can experience the stress-relieving benefits of this integrative therapy. Learn more about deep breathing on page 109.

Guided imagery

Your imagination is a powerful thing, and it's already built into your brain and ready for you to use. Guided imagery involves forming mental images of places or situations you find relaxing, usually under the guidance of an instructor, in person or virtually. There are a variety of apps and online programs available to help you with guided imagery. If you want to kick it up a notch, you can use your digital device, smart TV or virtual reality (VR) headset to immerse yourself more fully in a visual experience. Learn more about guided imagery on page 113 and virtual reality on page 216.

Meditation

At its core, meditation is a practice of focusing your attention on something that helps you achieve a state of physical relaxation, mental calmness and psychological balance. Maybe your focus is on your breathing, as you inhale and exhale, or on a specific word that you're repeating. Or maybe you meditate by taking a moment of gratitude before you sit down at your desk. Learn more about meditation on page 148.

As with guided imagery, you can also go high-tech with meditation. Download a meditation app on your digital device or receive real-time feedback from a headband that measures your brain waves. Apps typically charge a small monthly fee, while headbands may cost more up front. If it works for you, it may be an investment worth making, but it's not necessary.

Pilates

With nothing more than a mat and a YouTube video, you can practice Pilates as an integrative technique for both physical activity and stress relief, as well as other health and wellness benefits. If Pilates is new for you, talk to your doctor about it and get guidance from an instructor first. Learn more about Pilates on page 170.

Positive thinking

How you view the world around you and the everyday events in your life can make a significant difference in your overall well-being — and changing your thoughts costs you nothing. Learn about positive thinking and how you can use it to reframe your thoughts on pages 40 and 41.

Progressive muscle relaxation

Tensing and relaxing each of your muscle groups in sequence can help you find — and release — tension in your body. Learn more about progressive muscle relaxation on page 179.

Qigong

A Chinese medicine practice that generally combines meditation, relaxation, physical movement and breathing exercises, qigong is designed to restore and maintain balance. Learn how qigong represents a type of integrative physical activity that can promote health and wellness on page 186.

Spirituality

No matter how you experience spirituality, finding a way to connect with yourself and others, develop your personal value system, and search for meaning in life are all ways you can improve your wellness and quality of life. Learn more about spirituality on page 42.

Tai chi

Tai chi is a self-paced mind-body intervention that involves performing a series of postures or movements in a slow, graceful manner while practicing deep breathing. Tai chi requires no special equipment and can be done anywhere — indoors or outside, alone or in a group class.

Although you can watch online videos and read books about tai chi, consider seeking guidance from a qualified tai chi instructor to gain the full benefits and learn proper techniques. In addition, it's important to talk to your healthcare team first before trying tai chi — although it's generally safe, people with certain conditions may need to take extra precautions. Learn more about tai chi on page 209.

Yoga

Offering benefits for both physical and mental health, yoga involves performing a series of postures and controlled breathing exercises designed to promote a more flexible body and a calm mind. As you move through poses that require balance and concentration, you're encouraged to focus less on your busy day and more on the moment.

Although you can learn yoga from books and videos, beginners usually find it helpful to learn with an instructor. Speaking of beginners, if you are new to yoga, talk to your healthcare team first. Yoga is generally safe for most healthy people when it's practiced under the guidance of a trained instructor, but in some situations, yoga may pose risks. Learn more about yoga on page 218.

PARTNERING WITH YOUR HEALTHCARE TEAM

Some people are hesitant to discuss complementary therapies and holistic health approaches with their doctors, pharmacists or other members of their healthcare teams. Maybe you find yourself in this camp. Perhaps you're worried your healthcare team won't understand or will dismiss your desire to try unconventional treatments. But most medical professionals are well aware that complementary products and practices are highly popular, and they want to help their patients use these therapies safely and effectively.

Additionally, as evidence for many holistic therapies grows, more and more medical professionals are integrating these therapies into conventional medical care. Often, primary care doctors and nurses are well positioned to look at their patients' health with an eye toward quality of life.

Mutually beneficial

Discussing your interests and preferences with your healthcare team can help you determine which holistic methods might work best to keep you healthy or speed your recovery from illness or surgery.

At the same time, it helps your healthcare team to know what complementary therapies, herbs or supplements you're considering or using already. This way they can monitor your vital signs and lab results for any potential complications or interactions with prescription drugs you might be taking. Some herbs and supplements can also trigger allergies or digestive issues.

It also helps to be detailed. For example, if you're going to try massage, tell your healthcare team what type of massage you're interested in. Not all massages are the same. While Swedish or acupressure massages are quite gentle, Rolfing involves greater tissue manipulation and may not be for everybody. Similarly, certain yoga positions may not be appropriate if you have glaucoma or a back problem.

Make your own clinical trial

Consider each time you try a new therapy as a research trial with you — the patient — as an N of 1, or the sole participant. This means having a clear idea at the outset of what you are expecting the therapy to do and keeping a neutral attitude toward the end results.

Be specific. Saying "I want my arthritis pain to improve" is good, but it's better to describe your objective in detail: "My current pain is most noticeable in my knees and most days the pain level is pretty high, say an 8 out of 10. I want to reduce that level to a 4 or 5."

Start the therapy and then reassess those same symptoms. If they've improved, great. It doesn't mean for certain that it's because of the

236   Mayo Clinic Guide to Holistic Health

> # When it comes to your health, you want to make sure you're basing your decisions on trusted and credible information.

therapy, but it gives you a stronger reason to continue using that therapy. If you don't see any benefit, it may mean that you are not a "responder" to that particular therapy, and you may want to work with your healthcare team to try a different therapy.

If you're trying a new supplement, consider talking to your care team about doing some basic blood or urine tests to check for any unexpected side effects before you embark on long-term use of the supplement.

Work together

Although holistic approaches are becoming more widely accepted, some medical professionals may remain skeptical about certain practices and question their efficacy. Western medicine relies heavily on research studies that produce consistent and measurable results to identify safe and effective treatments. However, many holistic approaches rely on a whole-person approach to health and encompass many variables, making them challenging to study in a research setting. Often what works for one person may not work for another. Therefore, it's difficult to draw conclusions that can become part of an approved set of guidelines for physicians.

You may need to work with your healthcare team to find some middle ground. For example, if you want to try acupuncture for chronic pain, you might show them the latest research or an acupuncture page from the National Center for Complementary and Integrative Health.

Of course, you don't need permission from your care team to try different therapies. Many people take the best recommendations from their care team and then pursue other therapies on their own. But even if your care team isn't familiar enough with acupuncture, for example, to endorse it, they can at least make sure there is no strong medical reason for you not to try it.

Look for practitioners or healthcare centers that use holistic or integrative medicine

A growing number of hospitals and research institutions are adding integrative medicine departments to their organizations. For example, Mayo Clinic lists information on the integrative and holistic practices it offers on its website. You can search online for an integrative medicine department or practice near you.

FINDING HIGH-QUALITY RESEARCH

When it comes to your health, you want to make sure you're basing your decisions on trusted and credible information. Many websites, mobile apps and print publications provide health information, but not all of them are trustworthy. So where do you find reliable information?

A good place to start is government agency websites, such as the National Institutes of Health or the Centers for Disease Control and

FINDING A QUALIFIED PRACTITIONER

When seeking out a holistic medicine practitioner, be as careful and thorough as when searching for any other medical professional. Here are some tips drawn from the National Center for Complementary and Integrative Health.

Ask trusted sources
Your primary healthcare team, nearby hospitals or medical schools, professional organizations, state regulatory agencies or licensing boards, or even your health insurance provider may be helpful. And don't forget friends and family, who may have firsthand experience with a local therapist or practitioner specializing in an area you're interested in. See page 244 for a list of additional resources.

Do your homework
Find out as much as you can about any potential practitioner, including their education, training, licensing and certifications. Keep in mind that there is no standardized national system for credentialing complementary health practitioners. State governments are responsible for deciding what credentials practitioners must have to work in that state. Such credentials vary widely from state to state and from discipline to discipline.

Make introductions
Make sure the practitioner you choose is willing to work with other members of your healthcare team, such as your primary care doctor or

238 Mayo Clinic Guide to Holistic Health

Prevention, and well-respected hospitals and universities. Professional associations and nonprofit organizations dedicated to patient advocacy can often be valuable resources as well. Evidence-based studies that have been published in medical journals are also credible sources of health information, but not always free of charge. And let's face it — they're not always easy to interpret. Here are some pointers for evaluating clinical studies.

Terms to understand

As you've read through this book, you likely noticed terms such as "randomized controlled trial," "placebo" and "systematic reviews." What do these terms mean and how do they relate to your decision-making process?

specialist, as needed. Tell all your healthcare providers about the complementary approaches you use and about all the practitioners who are treating you. For safe, coordinated care, it's important for all the professionals involved in your health to communicate and cooperate.

Share information

Explain all your health conditions to the practitioner and find out about their training and experience in working with people who have your conditions. Choose a practitioner who understands how to work with people with your specific needs, even if general well-being is your goal. And remember that health conditions can affect the safety of complementary approaches; for example, if you have glaucoma, some yoga poses may not be safe for you.

Check insurance coverage

Don't assume that your health insurance will cover the practitioner's services. Ask your health insurance provider before getting treatment. Insurance plans differ greatly in what complementary health approaches they cover. If they do cover a particular approach, restrictions may apply.

Follow up with yourself

After your first visit, assess the care you received. Decide if this practitioner is right for you and the treatment plan is reasonable. It's OK to try a few different practitioners to find the best fit for you.

Tool kit **239**

You've likely also noticed sections that have highlighted research from "a small study," or research that lasted for a brief period. In these cases, it's noted that the therapy being discussed needs more research. What does that mean? Here are some key concepts and terms to know.

Clinical studies
Clinical studies are those that involve human beings — not animals. They're usually preceded by studies conducted in animals that demonstrate safety and effectiveness.

There are two major types of clinical studies.
- In an **observational study**, participants are simply observed and no treatment is given.
- In an **interventional study**, also known as a clinical trial, a treatment is given and monitored to learn if it works and if it's safe.

Rigorous clinical studies strive to control as many variables as possible. Variables are all the factors that can affect an outcome. Variables are many and not always known, but age and sex are two common examples. Ideally, a well-designed study leads to a significant amount of detailed data that shows how safe — and how helpful — a treatment may be.

In general, the larger the study, the better. When a study involves several hundred people or more — especially if it lasts over several months or years — it gains a wider perspective and more credibility.

How the study is performed also is key. Prospective double-blind studies that have been carefully controlled, randomized and published in peer-reviewed journals are the gold standard.

Randomized controlled trials
In this type of clinical study, participants are usually divided randomly into two groups. One group receives the treatment being studied, while the other group receives a placebo treatment.

Randomly assigning participants to one of two groups is done to ensure that participants with certain characteristics don't all end up in the same group. Randomly assigning participants is also a way to help balance the unique characteristics of the participants.

The first group receives the treatment under investigation. The second group is the control group. People in the control group may receive standard treatment, no treatment or an inactive substance called a placebo (see "The placebo effect" on opposite page).

Double-blind studies
Blinding a study is a lot like it sounds. In double-blind studies, neither the researchers nor the participants know who is receiving the active

240   Mayo Clinic Guide to Holistic Health

THE PLACEBO EFFECT

A placebo is a substance or therapy that appears to be a real medical treatment but isn't. A placebo could be a pill, a shot or some other type of false treatment. Often, a placebo is a sugar solution without any active ingredients, disguised to look like the pill or treatment it's trying to mimic.

What researchers have discovered is that people who think they're getting a real medicine when it's really just a placebo sometimes get better. This remarkable and quite real benefit is called the *placebo effect*, and it's a good example of how our minds and beliefs can affect our bodies. When you expect your physical symptoms to improve, they often do — even though you may not be doing or taking anything different.

Improvement due to the placebo effect is still improvement, and that's always welcome. But it's important to remember that for many health conditions, there are often treatments that work better than placebo treatments. That's why it's important to test all potential treatments to find out what works best for you.

treatment or the placebo. This type of study is also known as double-blind masking.

Prospective studies
Prospective studies are forward-looking. Researchers establish criteria for participants to follow and then measure or describe the results. Results from these studies are usually more reliable than retrospective study results.

Retrospective studies
The opposite of prospective studies, retrospective studies involve looking at past data, which leaves room for error in interpretation.

Peer-reviewed journals
These journals publish only articles that have been reviewed by an independent panel of medical experts. The review is usually anonymous, and the reviewers usually aren't paid. Browsing a journal's website — the "About" page, for example — can tell you more about the way they accept, review and publish researchers' manuscripts.

What to look for

When you're evaluating research on a particular therapy, look for clinical studies that involve human beings, not animals. Mice and humans have many genes in common, but a mouse is still not a human. Also check to see how the study was conducted and how many participants were involved.

Importantly, ask yourself if the research applies to you. For example, Mayo Clinic has conducted studies to see if ginseng can lessen fatigue in people who have had cancer. For these studies, the ginseng was obtained from a specific grower to help ensure that each capsule contained the same amount of active ingredients. In this case, ginseng helped those in the study group feel less fatigued. But that doesn't necessarily mean ginseng will have the same effect for you. If you're not buying the same type of ginseng and you're not a cancer survivor, you may not see the same results.

When looking at research, seek out not only high-quality studies but also studies that you can relate to based on your health profile and your goals for using the therapy.

The three D's

When looking for information on holistic health or a particular product or therapy, chances are you can find plenty of information — likely more than you need — on the internet. The internet offers a virtually limitless supply of information on all sorts of complementary and integrative treatments. But it's also one of the greatest sources of misinformation. As you're doing your homework, weed out the good information from the bad. To do that, use the three D's:

- **Dates** Check the creation or update date for each article. If you don't see a date, don't assume the article is recent. Older material may be outdated and may not include recent findings.
- **Documentation** Who operates the site? Are qualified health professionals creating and reviewing the information? Are references listed? Is advertising clearly identified?
- **Double-check** Visit several health websites and compare the information they offer. If you can't find supporting evidence to back up the claims of a holistic health product, be skeptical. And before you follow any advice you read on the internet, check with your healthcare team for guidance.

Bottom line: If what you read sounds too good to be true, it probably is. Make an effort to seek out additional information from a reliable, authoritative source, and talk with your doctor or another trusted healthcare professional.

Healthy habits have a powerful ripple effect.

TRANSFORMING YOUR HEALTH AND YOUR FUTURE

As you move forward in your wellness journey and consider ways that holistic practices can play a role in your health, think about the things you can do each day to enhance your well-being. Think of the basics that you learned about at the beginning of this book: sleep, exercise, nutrition, stress management, social support, purpose and meaning, and a connection to nature. What do you do each day to support your wellness in these areas? From eating whole foods and exercising regularly to meditating and spending time outdoors, every effort you make to improve your overall physical and mental health helps not just you but also your family and even your community.

Healthy habits have a powerful ripple effect. Look around to see what you can do to integrate the best complementary practices with the best of conventional medicine to achieve a lifetime of health and wellness.

additional resources

Following is a list of additional resources related to the topics covered in this book. Many of these are professional association websites, but they often include pages dedicated to consumers and patients, as well as search functions for finding local practitioners.

Academic Consortium for Integrative Medicine & Health
www.imconsortium.org

American Academy of Medical Acupuncture
www.medicalacupuncture.org

American Academy of Osteopathy
www.academyofosteopathy.org

American Association of Acupuncture and Oriental Medicine
www.aaaomonline.org

American Association of Naturopathic Physicians
www.naturopathic.org

American Botanical Council
https://abc.herbalgram.org

American Chiropractic Association
www.acatoday.org

American College of Lifestyle Medicine
https://lifestylemedicine.org

244   Mayo Clinic Guide to Holistic Health

American Holistic Health Association
https://ahha.org

American Massage Therapy Association
www.amtamassage.org

American Osteopathic Association
www.osteopathic.org

American Society of Clinical Hypnosis
www.asch.net

Association for Applied Psychophysiology and Biofeedback
www.aapb.org

Food and Drug Administration, Office of Dietary Supplement Programs
www.fda.gov/Food/DietarySupplements/default.htm

Healing Beyond Borders
www.healingbeyondborders.org

Mayo Clinic
www.mayoclinic.org

Mayo Clinic Connect
https://connect.mayoclinic.org

National Association for Holistic Aromatherapy
www.naha.org

National Cancer Institute, NIH
https://cam.cancer.gov

National Center for Complementary and Integrative Health
https://nccih.nih.gov

National Center for Homeopathy
www.homeopathic.org

ParkRx
www.parkrx.org

Additional resources   **245**

index

Academic Consortium for Integrative Medicine & Health, 14
acceptance, 16, 37, 44
acupressure, 140–141, 145, 195, 213, 214, 236
acupuncture, 64–72
  American Academy of Medical Acupuncture, 67
  for back pain, 64, 68, 70, 71, 72
  in cancer care, 66, 70–71
  conditions treated with, 64–65
  Evidence Based Acupuncture Project findings, 71, 72
  for fertility and pregnancy, 71
  for fibromyalgia, 70
  finding, working with a practitioner, 67–68
  for heart health, 71
  history of, 64
  at Mayo Clinic, 69
  National Certification Commission for Acupuncture and Oriental Medicine, 67
  for pain, 70
  practice and techniques of, 65
  preparing for treatment, 67
  research on, 69–72
  safety and risks of, 72
  for spinal stenosis, 71
  typical treatment session, 68–69
  Western and traditional Chinese views of, 65

adrenaline, 34, 35–36
alternative medicine, 17
Alzheimer's disease. *See also* dementia
  art therapy for, 89
  ginkgo for, 122
  music for, 163–165
  nutrition and, 31
  sauna use for, 199
  stress and, 36
ambient therapy, 48
animal-assisted services, 52, 73–79
  for chronic illness coping skills, 75
  facility dogs, 79
  for heart health, 74
  for improved quality of life, 74
  Mayo Clinic's Caring Canines, 73, 76–77
  Mayo Clinic's facility dogs program, 77
  research on, 74–75
  service dogs, 79
  for stress management, 74
  therapy dogs, 78
  therapy mini horse, 78
  tips for volunteering one's dog, 75, 77
anti-inflammatory properties and effects
  of acupuncture, 70
  of cryotherapy, 107
  of exercise, 21
  of foods and spices, 29, 31, 121, 122
  of sauna use, 199
  of vitamin D, 160
antioxidant properties and effects
  of aromatherapy, 81
  of cryotherapy, 107

of foods, 29, 30
of herbs and supplements, 121, 122
of sauna use, 190
of vitamin C, 160
of vitamin D, 160
antiviral properties and effects, 29, 156
anxiety
aromatherapy for, 84, 85
biofeedback for, 96
cannabis and cannabinoids for,
101–102
deep breathing for, 111
guided imagery for, 115
hypnotherapy for, 135
meditation and mindfulness for, 154
progressive muscle relaxation for, 180
psychedelics for, 185
Reiki for, 195
aromatherapy, 80–85
for anxiety, 84, 85
common scents used for relaxation, 81
for fatigue, 84, 85
finding a practitioner, 82
history of, 81
for labor pain and anxiety, 84
at Mayo Clinic, 83
National Association for Holistic
Aromatherapy, 82
for pain, 84
practice and techniques of, 80–82
research on, 84–85
safety and side effects of, 85
for sleep, 84–85
arrhythmia, 71
art therapy, 86–89
affordability of, 233
benefits of, 87–88
for brain-related disorders, 89
in cancer care, 89
history of, 87
at Mayo Clinic, 86
research on, 89
types of, 88–89
arthritis, 50–51
biofeedback for, 97
cryotherapy for, 107
hot tubs and warm pools for, 131

naturopathy for, 169
osteoarthritis, 64, 70, 72, 119, 144,
169, 215
rheumatoid arthritis, 53, 72, 97, 107,
144, 169
assessments and goal-setting
connection with nature, 229
emotional well-being, 228
general health, 227
health goals, 230–231
asthma, 96, 111, 154, 200
Ayurveda, 13, 99, 139, 148, 151

B

baby boomers, 55
back pain
acupuncture for, 64, 68, 70, 71, 72
biofeedback for, 96
cryotherapy for, 107
massage for, 141, 144
Pilates for, 171, 172
Rolfing for, 197, 198
sedentary lifestyles and, 22
spinal manipulation for, 202, 203,
206–207, 208
tui na for, 215
yoga for, 219
Bauer, Brent A., 43, 120, 214
Benzo, Roberto P., 12–13, 17, 149, 150,
152–153, 155
biofeedback, 90–97
for arthritis, 97
for asthma, 96
benefits of, 90–91
for chronic pain, 96
equipment, 92, 94–95
finding a practitioner, 92–93
for headache, 96
at home, 92–93
laws and regulations for, 93
at Mayo Clinic, 94–95
research on, 96–97
safety and risks of, 97
for stress and anxiety, 96
types of, 91

Index **247**

biofeedback continued
    typical treatment session, 91–92
    wearable devices, 92–93, 94–95
**Biofeedback Certification Institute
    of America**, 93
biophilic environments, 48–49
blood pressure
    deep breathing for, 112
    meditation and mindfulness for, 154
    naturopathy for, 169
    progressive muscle relaxation for, 180
    tui na for, 215
    yoga for, 222
Borkenhagen, Lynn, 86, 87
breathing, deep, 109–112
    affordability of, 234
    for anxiety, 111
    for asthma, 111
    benefits of, 111
    for blood pressure, 112
    chest breathing, 109
    diaphragmatic breathing tips, 109–110
    for insomnia, 112
    for nausea and vomiting, 111
    for pain, 111
    research on, 111–112
    safety and risks of, 112
    types of, 109–110

C

caffeine, 26, 28, 67
cancer care
    acupuncture in, 66, 70–71
    art therapy in, 89
    complementary therapies and, 55
    guided imagery in, 115
    massage therapy in, 146
    meditation and mindfulness in, 154
    progressive muscle relaxation in, 180
    reflexology in, 192
    Reiki in, 115
    Society for Integrative Oncology, 55
    tai chi in, 212
    wellness and, 51–55, 58–59
    yoga in, 222

cannabis and cannabinoids, 98–105
    for anxiety, 102
    CBD, 98, 100, 102, 104–105
    Cesamet, 101
    definitions and terminology, 98–99
    endocannabinoid system of human
        body, 100
    Epidiolex, 101, 104, 105
    for epilepsy, 101, 105
    history of, 98
    marijuana, 98, 99, 100
    Marinol, 101
    for multiple sclerosis, 101, 102
    for pain, 101
    for PTSD, 102
    regulation of, 100–101
    research on, 101–102
    safety and risks of, 103–105
    Syndros, 101
    THC, 98, 100, 101, 104, 105
Chinese medicine, traditional, 13, 119, 122,
    139, 167, 188. *See also* acupressure;
    acupuncture; qigong; tai chi; *tui na*
chiropractic. *See* spinal manipulation
compassion, 16, 37, 44
cortisol, 34–36, 82, 88, 154, 181, 211, 218
costs and budgets, holistic health and,
    233–235
COVID-19
    guided imagery and, 115
    homeopathy and, 129
    mind-body techniques and, 156, 222
    pandemic's impact on health and
        wellness, 18–19, 132
    pandemic's impact on healthcare
        professionals, 154, 217
    pandemic's impact on social
        connectedness, 38
    in people with obesity, 108
    sauna use and, 200
Croghan, Ivana T., 94–95
cryotherapy, 106–108
    for chronic low back pain, 107
    for heart health, 107
    history of, 106
    for mental health, 108
    for multiple sclerosis, 107

248   Mayo Clinic Guide to Holistic Health

practice and techniques of, 106–107
research on, 107–108
for rheumatoid arthritis, 107
safety and risks of, 108
for weight loss, 108
Cutshall, Susanne M., 83, 117, 118, 194
cytokines, 13, 21, 82

D

DASH diet, 31
Davis, Chip, 48
deep breathing. *See* breathing, deep
dementia. *See also* Alzheimer's disease
animal-assisted services for, 75
art therapy for, 87
ginkgo for, 122
loneliness and, 38
massage for, 144
music for, 165
nutrition and, 31
reflexology for, 192
sauna use for, 199, 200
stress and, 36
depression
animal-assisted services for, 74, 75, 79
aromatherapy for, 82, 84
art therapy for, 87, 89
cryotherapy for, 108
deep breathing for, 111
exercise for, 22, 23
healing touch for, 117
herbs and supplements for, 122, 123
massage therapy for, 139, 140, 144
meditation and mindfulness for,
154–155, 157
mind-body techniques for, 154
Pilates for, 171
progressive muscle relaxation for, 180
psychedelics for, 182, 183, 185
reflexology for, 191, 192
Reiki for, 193
tai chi for, 210, 212
yoga for, 220, 221, 222
diabetes, 13
exercise for, 21

herbs and supplements for, 121, 122, 123
integrative medicine and, 14
nutrition and, 32
reflexology for, 192
sleep deprivation and, 26
stress management for, 36
tai chi for, 212
Do, Alexander, 188, 189, 211

E

emotional wellness, 16
exercise, 21–25
aerobic fitness, 23–24
anti-inflammatory effects of, 21
balance training, 24
benefits of, 21–23
core exercises, 24
flexibility and stretching, 24–25
heart and lung health benefits of, 22–23
insulin benefits of, 21
mental and emotional well-being, 23
for new mothers, 52
risks of being sedentary, 22
sleep and, 27
strength training, 24
types of, 23–25
weight and muscle mass benefits of, 21

F

fertility and pregnancy, 71
fibromyalgia, 14, 53, 232
acupuncture for, 70
hypnosis for, 134
massage therapy for, 143, 144
music for, 165
tai chi for, 210
warm water and sauna use for, 132, 200
fight-or-flight response, 34, 36, 218–219
Fitzgerald, William, 190
forgiveness, 37, 43, 44
friendship, 17, 38, 42. *See also* social
connectedness
Fuehrer, Debbie L., 137

G

gratitude, 16, 17, 27, 35, 37, 43, 44, 60, 234
guided imagery, 113–115
    affordability of, 234
    for anxiety, 115
    for before and after surgery, 114
    in cancer care, 115
    color imagery, 114
    for enhancing performance, 115
    for pain, 115
    practice and techniques of, 113–114
    research on, 114–115
    for sleep, 115

H

Hahnemann, Samuel, 126
Hauschulz, Jennifer L., 142–143, 145, 190, 191
headache
    acupuncture for, 64, 70
    biofeedback for, 96
    CoQ10 for, 121
    massage therapy for, 141, 143
    progressive muscle relaxation for, 181
    psychedelics for, 183
    Reiki for, 193
    spinal manipulation for, 202, 204, 206, 207, 208
    yoga for, 221
healing touch, 116–118
    history of, 116–117
    at Mayo Clinic, 117
    research on, 118
    typical session, 118
Healing Touch International, 116–117
healthcare team, talking about holistic health with, 236–238
heart health
    acupuncture for, 71
    animal-assisted services for, 74
    cryotherapy for, 107
    exercise for, 22–23
    hot tubs and warm pools for, 132
    massage therapy for, 144

    meditation and mindfulness for, 154
    naturopathy for, 169
herbs and supplements, 119–125
    coenzyme Q10 (CoQ10), 121
    FDA and regulations of, 125
    fish oils, 119
    flaxseed and flaxseed oil, 123
    garlic, 121
    ginger, 124
    ginkgo, 121–122
    ginseng, 122
    glucosamine and chondroitin, 119–120
    history of, 119
    iron, 124
    at Mayo Clinic, 120
    melatonin, 120–121
    safety and risks of, 124–125
    saw palmetto, 121
    St. John's Wort, 123
    turmeric and curcumin, 122
    valerian, 123
    zinc, 124
high blood pressure. *See* blood pressure
Holmes, Ben, 204, 206, 207
Homeopathic Academy of Naturopathic Physicians, 128
homeopathy, 126–130
    finding and working with a practitioner, 128–129
    history of, 126
    "homeopathic aggravation," 130
    nanomedicine and, 129
    products, practices and techniques, 126–128
    regulation of, 127
    research on, 129
    safety and risks of, 130
hot tubs and warm pools, 131–135.
    See also saunas
    for arthritis, 131
    for fibromyalgia, 132
    for heart health, 132
    history of, 131, 133
    "hot tub lung," 132
    Mayo Clinic's Rejuvenate Spa, 133, 199–200
    medical spas, 131

250   Mayo Clinic Guide to Holistic Health

research on, 131–132
safety and risks of, 132–133
for sleep and mood, 132
Huang, Linda, 119–120, 121–122, 123, 124, 125
Hurt, Ryan T., 174–176
hypnotherapy, 134–138
American Society of Clinical Hypnosis, 136
for anxiety, 135
for chronic pain, 135
conditions treated with, 134–135
finding a therapist, 136
at Mayo Clinic, 137
for postoperative pain, 135
research on, 135
safety and risks of, 137–138
typical therapy session, 136–137
hypothalamus, 34, 80

I

illness
cancer treatment and wellness, 51–54, 58–59
as catalyst for personal growth, 58–60
examples of holistic wellness during, 52–53, 58–59
medications and, 56–58
tips for taking charge of your health, 59
wellness during, 50–59
Ingham, Eunice, 190
insomnia, 27
acupuncture for, 66
aromatherapy for, 84, 85
cannabis and, 98, 102
deep breathing for, 112
homeopathy for, 129
hypnosis for, 137
medications and supplements for, 120–121
reflexology for, 192
Reiki for, 193
screens and, 27
yoga for, 218, 220, 221
integrative medicine, 14, 15, 17, 237–238

Academic Consortium for Integrative Medicine & Health, 14
Mayo Clinic Integrative Medicine and Health, 14
intellectual wellness, 16
introverts, 39

J

Jacobson, Edmund, 179

K

Kopecky, Stephen, 18–19, 35, 57, 59

L

Larson, Jean, 47
life energy, 116, 186, 188, 209, 211
loneliness, 38, 39, 74, 79, 154. *See also* social connectedness

M

Mallory, Molly J., 66, 67, 68, 70, 71
marijuana. *See* cannabis and cannabinoids
massage therapy, 139–147
for aging, 144
benefits of, 139–140
in cancer care, 146
cranial massage, 141
deep tissue massage, 140
for fibromyalgia, 144
for heart health, 144
history of, 139
hot stone massage, 141
lymphatic drainage massage, 141
at Mayo Clinic, 145
for mental health and wellness, 144
for pain relief, 142, 143–144
reflexology, 141
research on, 142–144, 146
safety and risks of, 146–147

Index   **251**

massage therapy continued
    shiatsu massage, 139, 140
    sports massage, 140
    Swedish massage, 140
    Thai massage, 141
    trigger point massage, 141
    types of, 140–141
    typical massage session, 141
    for workplace stress management, 146
Mayo Clinic Integrative Medicine and Health, 14
meaning. *See* spirituality and purpose
medications
    balancing wellness and, 56–57
    opioids, 56, 57, 66, 69, 83, 101, 143
    questions to ask about new medications, 58
    taking too much, 56
    varying effects of, 57
meditation and mindfulness, 148–157
    affordability of, 234
    for anxiety, depression and stress, 154
    for asthma, 154
    being present, 152
    benefits of, 152–153
    body scan meditation, 149
    in cancer care, 154
    guided meditation, 149–150
    for heart health and blood pressure, 154
    history of, 148, 151
    for immune function, 156
    for irritable bowel syndrome, 156
    love and kindness meditation, 150
    mantra meditation, 150
    at Mayo Clinic, 12, 149, 155
    mindfulness tips, 151–152
    practice and techniques of, 149–152
    research on, 152–156
    sitting meditation, 149
    for sleep problems, 154
    walking meditation, 149
Mentgen, Jane, 116
metabolic disorders, 169, 175, 200
Metchnikov, Ilya, 173–174
Metzger, Abbey K., 83, 196
migraine. *See* headache

mindfulness. *See* meditation and mindfulness
Mosley, William, 59
multiple sclerosis, 52, 101, 102, 107, 144, 175, 192
multivitamins, 158–162
    discovery of vitamins, 158
    foods vs. supplements, 161
    safety and risks of, 161–162
    vitamin B-1, 158–159
    vitamin B-3, 159
    vitamin B-6, 159–160
    vitamin B-12, 160
    vitamin C, 160
    vitamin D, 160–161
muscle relaxation, progressive, 179–181
    for anxiety, 180
    in cancer care, 180
    for headaches, 181
    for high blood pressure, 180
    history of, 179
    practice and techniques of, 179
    research on, 179–181
    for stress management, 180–181
music therapy, 163–166
    for Alzheimer's disease, 165
    for autism, 165
    benefits of, 163–164
    for cerebral palsy, 166
    for exercise performance, 165
    for pain, 165
    practice and techniques of, 164
    research on, 164–166
    safety and risks of, 166
    for stroke, 165

N

National Center for Complementary and Integrative Health, 82, 237, 238
nature, connection with, 45–49
    ambient therapy, 48
    benefits of, 46–47
    biophilic environments, 48–49
    shinrin-yoku (forest bathing), 47
    tips for, 47–48

252   Mayo Clinic Guide to Holistic Health

naturopathy, 167–169
  for arthritis, 169
  benefits of, 167
  for blood pressure and weight loss, 169
  history of, 167
  naturopathic physicians, 168
  practices and techniques of, 168
  for reducing risk of heart disease, 169
  research on, 169
  traditional naturopaths, 168
neck pain
  acupuncture for, 64, 70, 72
  massage for, 144
  qigong for, 189
  Rolfing for, 197
  spinal manipulation for, 202, 203, 206,
    207, 208
nutrition, 28–34
  alcohol, 30
  carbohydrates, 29
  DASH diet, 31
  fats, 30
  healthy habits and tips, 32–34
  Mediterranean diet, 31, 33
  mindful eating, 32
  protein and dairy, 29–30
  sweets, 30
  vegetables and fruits, 29

O

opioids, 56, 57, 66, 70, 83, 101, 143
optimism, 17, 40–41, 59, 89, 218
osteopathy. *See* spinal manipulation

P

pain. *See also* arthritis; back pain;
    headache; neck pain
  acupuncture for, 70
  aromatherapy for, 84, 85
  biofeedback for, 96
  cancer pain, 71, 89, 144
  cannabis and cannabinoids for, 101
  deep breathing for, 111

  guided imagery for, 115
  hypnotherapy for, 135
  labor pain, 84
  massage therapy for, 142, 143–144
  music therapy for, 165
  postoperative pain, 135
  Reiki for, 195
  virtual reality for, 217
Palmer, David, 202
Parkinson's disease, 31, 47, 140, 175, 187,
    210, 212
phobias, 135, 216–217. *See also* anxiety
physical wellness, 16
Pilates, 170–172
  affordability of, 234
  for back pain, 171
  finding an instructor, 172
  history of, 170
  for mental health, 171
  practice and techniques of, 170–171
  research on, 171–172
  safety and risks of, 172
  for scoliosis, 172
  for strength, balance and endurance,
    171
  for stroke, 172
placebo effect, 241
polypharmacy, 56
pools, warm. *See* hot tubs and warm
    pools
positive thinking, 40–41, 59, 60, 89, 218,
    234
post-traumatic stress disorder (PTSD),
    102, 184–185, 216–217
prebiotics, 174–175, 176, 178
probiotics, 173–178
  bacterial strains of, 174
  benefits of, 174–175
  choosing a supplement, 176
  for diarrhea, 177
  in fermented foods, 176
  healthy microbiomes and, 175–176
  history of, 173–174
  for infants and children's health, 177
  in kefir, 174
  microplastics and, 177
  prebiotics and, 174–175, 176, 178

Index **253**

probiotics continued
    research on, 176–177
    safety, risks and side effects of, 177–178
    for ulcerative colitis, 177
progressive muscle relaxation. *See*
    muscle relaxation, progressive
pro-inflammatory properties and effects,
    13, 21, 82
psychedelics, 182–185
    in addiction treatment, 184
    ayahuasca, 182, 183, 184
    for depression and anxiety, 185
    history of, 183
    LSD, 182, 183
    MDMA (ecstasy), 183, 184–185
    from naturally occurring substances, 182
    for PTSD, 184–185
    regulation of, 182
    research on, 183–185
purpose. *See* spirituality and purpose

Q

qigong, 52, 186–189, 209–211, 218, 235
    affordability of, 235
    for chronic fatigue, 187
    finding a practitioner, 187
    history of, 186
    meditative elements of, 118
    for memory and cognition, 188
    for mobility and balance, 187
    for Parkinson's disease, 187
    research on, 187–188
    safety and risks of, 189
    science of, 188
    for strength and posture, 187
    styles of, 186

R

reflexology, 190–192
    benefits of, 191
    for cancer pain, 192
    in childbirth, 192
    history of, 190

Ingham method, 190–191
    at Mayo Clinic, 191
    for mental health, 192
    for multiple sclerosis, 192
    research on, 191–192
    Rwo Shur method, 190–191
Reiki, 17, 193–196
    in cancer treatment, 115
    finding a practitioner, 194
    history of, 193
    levels of training, 194
    at Mayo Clinic, 117, 195
    for pain and fatigue, 195
    practice and techniques of, 193
    research on, 195
    safety and risks of, 196
    for stress and anxiety, 195
    typical session, 194
research, finding high-quality, 239–242
rheumatoid arthritis, 53, 72, 97, 107,
    144, 169
Rolfing, 197–198
    history of, 197
    practice and techniques of, 197
    research on, 197–198
    safety and risks of, 198
    typical session, 197
Romine, Whitney, 73, 74, 75, 76–77

S

saunas, 199–201. *See also* hot tubs
    and warm pools
    benefits of, 199–200
    for common colds and asthma, 200
    for fibromyalgia, 200
    for healthy cognitive aging, 200
    history of, 199
    infrared saunas, 201
    Mayo Clinic's Rejuvenate Spa, 133,
    199–200
    for pneumonia, 200
    practice and techniques of, 199
    research on, 200
    for rheumatic conditions, 200
    safety and risks of, 201

self-talk, 41. *See also* positive thinking
sleep. *See also* insomnia
  aromatherapy for, 84–85
  exercise for, 27
  guided imagery for, 115
  historical accommodations for, 25
  hot tubs and warm pools for, 132
  medications and supplements for, 27
  meditation and mindfulness for, 154
  naps, 28
  purpose of, 26
  REM sleep, 25
  schedules, 26
  screens and, 27
  tips for better sleep, 26–28
sleep hygiene, 26
social connectedness, 38–42
  benefits of, 39–41
  friendship, 17, 38, 42
  introverts and, 39
  loneliness and, 38, 39
  optimism and, 40–41
  spirituality and, 45
  tips for building quality relationships, 42
social wellness, 16–17
Sood, Amit, 37
spinal manipulation, 202–208
  American Chiropractic Association,
    202, 206
  American Osteopathic Association,
    206
  back pain, 206–207
  chiropractic, 202–203
  finding a chiropractor, 206
  history of, 202
  holistic routines and, 204
  at Mayo Clinic, 206
  for migraines, 207
  osteopathy, 203–205
  research on, 206–207
  safety and risks of, 207–208
  typical chiropractor visit, 205–206
spinal stenosis, 71, 172
spiritual wellness, 16
spirituality and purpose, 16, 43–45
  affordability of, 235
  assessing and goal-setting, 229

benefits of, 43–44
health and, 45
nurturing relationships and, 45
stress management and, 37
tips for cultivating, 44
Still, Andrew, 203
stress management, 13–14, 16, 34–38
  animal-assisted services for, 74
  biofeedback for, 96
  during COVID-19 pandemic, 18
  exercise for, 23, 24–25
  fight-or-flight response, 34, 36, 218–219
  gratitude practice for, 35, 37
  during illness, 54
  massage therapy for, 146
  meditation and mindfulness for, 154
  modern stress, 34–36
  natural settings for, 35
  nutrition and, 27
  physiological responses to stress, 34
  prejudices and, 37
  principles for, 37
  progressive muscle relaxation for,
    180–181
  Reiki for, 195
  sensual engagement for, 35
  sleep and, 27, 28
  spirituality and, 37
  tips for, 35
  virtual reality for, 217

T

tai chi, 17, 209–212
  affordability of, 235
  for balance, 210
  beginner exercises, 211
  in cancer care, 212
  for COPD, 210–211
  during COVID-19 pandemic, 211
  for depression and mood, 212
  finding an instructor, 209
  history of, 209
  at Mayo Clinic, 211
  meditative elements of, 118
  for Parkinson's disease, 210

Index   **255**

tai chi continued
    for physical fitness, 210
    practice and techniques of, 209–210
    research on, 210–212
    safety, risks and side effects of, 212
    for strength, 210
    styles of, 209–210
    typical session, 210
Tilburt, Jon C., 15
tui na, 213–215
    AI-assisted *tui na*, 214
    in China, 213
    for dyspepsia, 215
    for high blood pressure, 215
    history of, 213
    for low back pain, 215
    for musculoskeletal and joint
        conditions, 215
    practice and techniques of, 213–214
    research on, 214–215

U

Usui, Mikao, 193

V

Vincent, Ann, 102–103
virtual reality, 216–217
    for pain, 217
    practice and techniques of, 216
    for PTSD and phobias, 217
    research on, 216–217
    safety and risks of, 217
    for stress management, 217
    VRET (virtual reality exposure
        therapy), 216–217

W

water, warm. *See* hot tubs and warm
    pools; saunas
wellness, maximizing, 16–17
Whiting, Jenna, 86–87

whole health, 15
Wilson, Edward O., 46

Y

yoga, 218–223
    affordability of, 235
    benefits of, 218–220
    for blood pressure, 222
    in cancer care, 222
    for headaches, 221
    history of, 218
    for IBS, 222
    for immune system health, 221–222
    meditative elements of, 118
    for overall wellness, 221
    practice and techniques of, 220–221
    research on, 221–222
    safety and risks of, 222–223

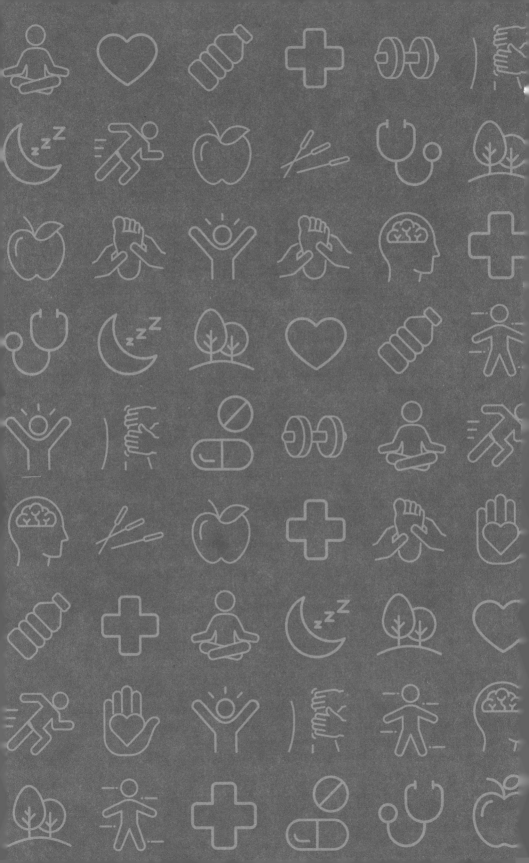